The Body Buddies

The Body Buddies

by Dr. Bernard Ernst and Jeanne Ernst

Coordinated by
Bernard Clendenin

Collier Books
A Division of
Macmillan Publishing Co., Inc.
New York

Collier Macmillan Publishers
London

Macmillan Publishing Co., Inc.
866 Third Avenue,
New York, N.Y. 10022
Collier Macmillan
Canada, Ltd.

Library of Congress Cataloging
in Publication Data
Ernst, Bernard.
    The body buddies.
    1. Exercise. 2. Diet. 3. Physical
fitness.   I.   Ernst, Jeanne, joint author.
II.   Title.
RA781. E76   613.7'1   79-303
ISBN 0-02-058750-3

First Printing 1979

Designed by James Udell

Printed in the United States of America

DEDICATION

To all of the viewers of our "Body Buddies"
television program and our family of friends
everywhere, who have been of immeasurable
help and encouragement.

We love you all.

Contents

ACKNOWLEDGMENTS

The list of people who have helped us along the way grows longer and longer as our efforts continue in the health and exercise field.

Putting together this book was not a singular feat, and we wish to thank all those who have contributed many hours of work, understanding, and support. In particular, the vision and patience of Bernard Clendenin was ever-present.

We especially want to mention the untiring efforts of Rollin Olson, producer, "Body Buddies"; Harold Moskowitz, literary agent; Terence Ford, photographer; Lionel Schaen, vice-president and general manager, RKO-KHJ TV, Los Angeles; Walt Baker, vice-president and program manager, RKO-KHJ TV; Dave Ryan, president, Nutrition Educators; Denis and Janet Walp, vice-presidents, Nutrition Educators; Golda Clendenin, Joel Kimmel, and Michael Wallack, M.D.

These exercises have been carefully chosen by Dr. Bernie and Jeanne Ernst to apply to beginners and advanced students. The photographs were designed to clearly illustrate how easy exercising can be and what results to expect by following a prescribed schedule that soon will become an invigorating, energy-producing routine.

By developing a positive mental attitude, you will:

- Feel more youthful

- Have a healthy life-style

- Find that beauty and exercise go hand in hand

SIX PRINCIPLES OF PHYSICAL FITNESS

1. **Regular Exercise**
2. **Proper Nutrition**
3. **Rest and Relaxation**
4. **Fresh Air and Sunshine**
5. **Positive Mental Attitude**
6. **Elimination of Dissipations**

DO'S AND DONT'S

1. Exhale on the effort, except when you compress the rib cage.
2. When doing standing exercises, always stand with legs apart, unlock knees, and tighten buttocks. This takes the stress off the lower back.
3. When doing any sit-ups always bend knees. This protects the lower back.
4. When doing exercises, try to pull the stomach in.
5. The fastest way to improve is to work against resistance. The number of times you do an exercise or the use of weights is considered resistance.
6. In the beginning your own body weight will be your resistance. To improve performance, add more repetitions or use weights.
7. To build a muscle, do slow, concentrated repetitions and use weights. To reduce an area, do repetitions at a fast pace.
8. Never bounce in stretching. Smooth, easy motions are best. Always hold a stretch for at least ten seconds. Never try to stretch too far. If it hurts, you are forcing the exercise.
9. Seventy-five percent of the stomach work is performed with the small of the back still on the floor. For example, in doing a sit-up (on your back, knees bent), almost all the work is put on your stomach muscles before your lower back leaves the floor.
10. Women will be more comfortable wearing a good support bra or a leotard that gives support. Wear clothing that is comfortable and not binding.
11. Men need to wear outfits that are not binding, are stretchable, and are non-restricting.

INTRODUCTION

"Try to lose some weight, improve your diet, get some regular exercise, and learn to relax."

How many times have I and other physicians given this basic common-sense advice to patients, and how rarely are these recommendations followed?

"I know you're right doctor, and I'll try," is the usual response, but at the time of the next annual physical the same habit patterns usually exist.

What is the problem? These recommendations are simple, inexpensive, do not require a prescription, are fun, there are no side effects, and the benefits can be considerable.

Achieving and maintaining a normal body weight in addition to improving one's appearance and self-esteem have been shown to reduce blood pressure, ameliorate diabetes for many individuals, reduce cholesterol and fat levels in the body, and lower the chances of getting degenerative arthritis, gout, and phlebitis. In addition, a person with normal weight can much more easily tolerate any surgical operation that might be necessary.

Weight reduction and exercise go hand in hand. An active individual can lose weight much more readily than a sedentary person given the same caloric intake. In addition, regular exercise has been shown to have benefits in alleviating depression, enhancing the efficiency and function of the heart, lungs, and circulatory system, and may reduce the chances of stroke and heart attack.

Getting out of shape and being overweight are problems that do not arise overnight or in a week or a month, and their correction requires a long-term steady solution. Fad crash diets and sudden vigorous exercise programs usually do not work in the long run and they have potential serious side effects.

In **The Body Buddies,** a common-sense, coordinated approach to exercise, weight loss, nutrition, and relaxation is described in a manner that is easy to follow, prudent, and that should have long-term permanent benefits both physically and mentally for those able to implement this program.

Michael Wallack, M.D.

Anatomy and Terminology

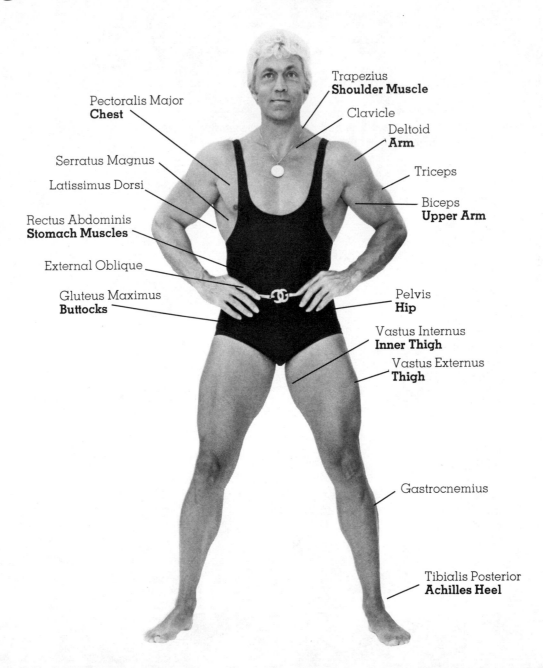

Pectoralis Major
Chest

Serratus Magnus

Latissimus Dorsi

Rectus Abdominis
Stomach Muscles

External Oblique

Gluteus Maximus
Buttocks

Trapezius
Shoulder Muscle

Clavicle

Deltoid
Arm

Triceps

Biceps
Upper Arm

Pelvis
Hip

Vastus Internus
Inner Thigh

Vastus Externus
Thigh

Gastrocnemius

Tibialis Posterior
Achilles Heel

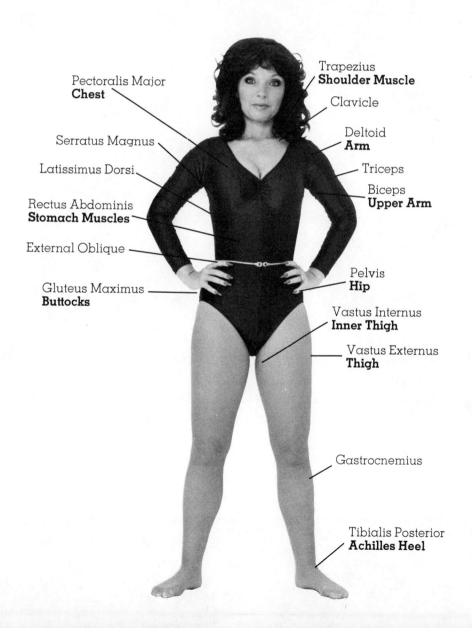

Pectoralis Major
Chest

Serratus Magnus

Latissimus Dorsi

Rectus Abdominis
Stomach Muscles

External Oblique

Gluteus Maximus
Buttocks

Trapezius
Shoulder Muscle

Clavicle

Deltoid
Arm

Triceps

Biceps
Upper Arm

Pelvis
Hip

Vastus Internus
Inner Thigh

Vastus Externus
Thigh

Gastrocnemius

Tibialis Posterior
Achilles Heel

Body Buddies Concepts

If your mind can make you sick, and it can, it can also make you well. Your mind is very powerful. If you let stresses and emotional upsets get to you, you can become physically sick. But you can also feed your mind positive thoughts about your health and your ability to meet the stresses of life.

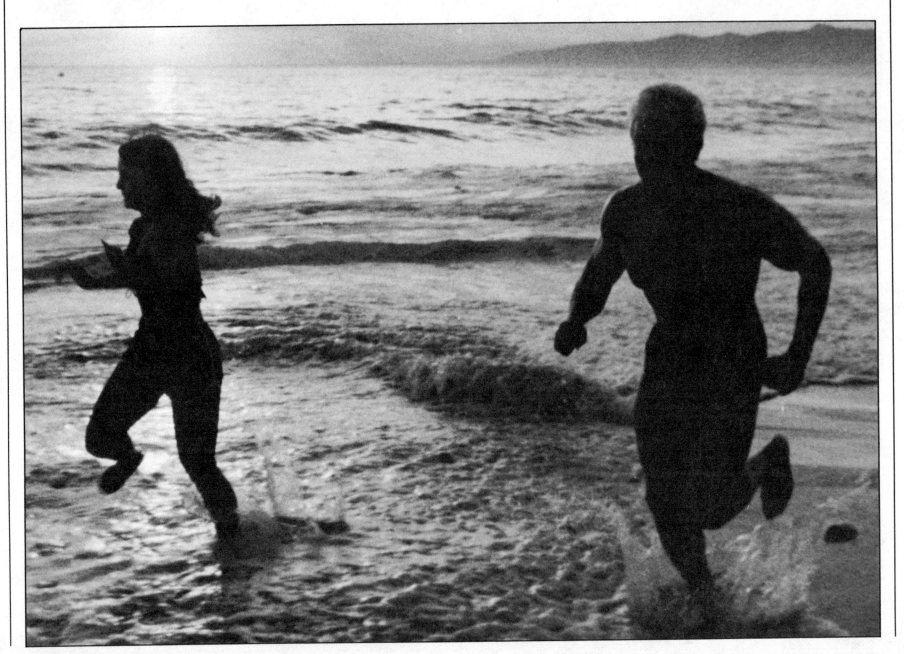

EXERCISE IS NOT A DIRTY WORD

There's something in the air. Step out your front door and watch joggers striding down the street, Frisbee advocates playing catch, basketballs being dribbled, executives hustling to keep racquetball and tennis appointments, health food stores and restaurants replacing familiar greasy spoons. "The times they are a-changing," Bob Dylan once declared, and now is the time to rise up off the couch and turn off the television. Commit yourself to being a participant and find a "body buddy" in the form of husband, wife, friend, or lover to engage in an exciting, invigorating, and satisfying program dedicated to fitness, health, and a happier life. Within weeks the familiar husband-wife litany, "We have nothing in common," will fade into oblivion. You'll feel better, look better, have greater self-esteem. The principles by which the Body Buddies live are simple in nature and follow the basic rules of common sense. These fitness principles include regular exercise, proper nutrition, rest and relaxation, fresh air and sunshine, a positive mental attitude, and the elimination of dissipations. If followed, they go a long way in reducing stress, anxiety, unhappiness, anger, and a poor self-image in daily life. The Body Buddies provide an example for those around them while creating a beautiful life-style for themselves.

Fitness is basically a question of attitude. We've been programmed with characterizations of the good life—dream houses with plush furnishings, limousines and sports cars, fine wines, gourmet foods, expensive cigars—which must be modified if we are to achieve our goals of fitness and health. Here are some hints to develop another approach to good living.

1. Try standing when you normally would sit.
2. Use the stairs instead of escalators and elevators.
3. Leave the car at home when going short distances. You can walk, jog, roller-skate, or bicycle.
4. Get outdoors more often.
5. Fill your refrigerator with healthful snacks.
6. Find someone to exercise with.
7. Exercise gradually and choose exercises you like or those that suit your goals.
8. Don't set impossible goals. Start exercising with a fifteen-minute time limit, rather than an hour or more.
9. Think positively.
10. Reward yourself. You deserve the best every day. Remember—don't reward yourself with food. That extra inch will make you uncomfortable.

The core idea of Body Buddies is "staying fit together." This does not imply that the same exercises must be practiced by both people. Do those exercises you each like individually. The concept here is to establish the goals of fitness and health around specific areas of interest. The goal statement helps to keep you moving in a positive direction. We're assuming you are in poor physical condition and have the desire to become fit. A good mental attitude is your guide in changing inertia into action. We're with you!

1 Body Buddies Concepts

BEGINNERS' CAUTIONS

In the exercise field, beginners are not so much novices as people who have not worked their muscles since high school or college. The eight-to-five office jobs and the misconception that relaxing is flaking out on the couch to watch TV or listen to music have caused muscles to grow soft and weak. In planning and determining a Body Buddies program of exercise and diet, we recommend consulting with your personal physician. Get a physical checkup—it can't hurt and it can definitely help.

After your doctor's approval, small goals should be established and short time periods set aside for exercising. Start with fifteen-minute exercise sessions. Always warm up prior to exercising. Use the warm-up techniques described in the chapters on Warming-up, Daily Dozens, or the section on Jogging.

You're a beginner. Don't try to do as much as someone who is already in good shape, such as your exercise instructor. What we're really saying is to bend over or touch or twist only as far as you are able. Don't overdo. It is easy to get sore muscles.

Each exercise has a starting position and a finishing position. From start to finish is considered one repetition. Thus, doing the same exercise ten times is called ten repetitions, or ten reps. We recommend beginners do ten reps per exercise and no more than twelve exercises per day.

When you exercise with a body buddy, do not try to compete with him/her, or even do the same exercises at the same time. It is important that you do the exercises that complement your specific goals. Before starting any session, be sure that you have sufficiently warmed up and conditioned your muscles. If you plan a program of jogging, begin with short distances and try to run on grassy surfaces.

Whichever exercise program you select, build up by gradually adding repetitions, distance, or both to your routine. Use the calendar in the book as an aid. As you start to achieve goals, pat yourself on the back, be proud of your efforts. So enjoy, take it easy, and you'll make it easy.

SEXUALITY AND EXERCISING

There really is a relationship between sexuality and exercising, you know. Being fit produces greater health, energy, body sensitivity, attractiveness, strength, awareness, and endurance. And these elements play an important role in sexuality. Think about it. Of course, it is impossible to make really accurate generalizations that could apply to every man or woman reading this book, or any other book regarding sexuality, and being "in shape" is not enough in itself to guarantee a healthy, happy relationship or even to start one. However, bear in mind the fact that being in a rundown condition as a result of alcohol, narcotics, smoking, improper nutrition, lack of essential vitamins, or lack of sleep will not make you the answer to a maiden's or gentleman's prayer, either in bed or out of it.

There is enough evidence around to prove that alcohol, sugar, and cigarettes decrease the sex hormones while robbing the body of essential nutrients and vitamins that provide the energy necessary to make love. Women are complaining about the infrequency of sex with men in their twenties and thirties—men who've dissipated themselves with the wrong kinds of food and too much alcohol.

The typical American starts the day poorly with the usual sweet roll and coffee (sugar and caffeine), then wonders why he feels tired a few hours later. A breakfast of pastry and coffee initially causes a sudden rise in blood sugar level. But the body reacts to too much sugar with chemical changes that lower blood sugar rapidly and cause fatigue. The problem is aggravated by high-carbohydrate lunches and dinners. By seven o'clock in the evening the energy factory has stopped producing. Our typical American is pooped. He collapses in front of the T.V. You can see how a person's sex life can easily deteriorate.

Any man or woman who begins an exercise program and takes care of him or herself by eating the proper kinds of food will increase sexual potency and lasting powers. Women have reported remarkable differences in the sexual performance of their husbands after they began jogging and cut out the energy-stealing foods.

As body buddies you can work toward a common fitness goal. Communicate your goals to your body buddy. A man's goal may be entirely different from a woman's. It's all a matter of the individual's needs and can be determined at the outset of the exercise program.

Sexuality can also be viewed as the radiance and beauty reflected in a healthy face and body—the change in attitude and positive image concept. Learn to like yourself. It enhances your personality and attracts people to you.

Body Buddies Concepts

BREATHING

The blood performs the two vital functions of taking in oxygen and giving off carbon dioxide in the lungs. These two functions occur simultaneously. The lungs are divided into many small air sacs called alveoli. Air drawn into the lungs enters the alveoli and comes into close contact with the blood vessels. When this contact occurs, the blood absorbs oxygen from the air and gives off its carbon dioxide.

The lungs themselves do not actively expand or contract; they only fill up partially. Consequently, they need help. Deep breathing exercises are valuable because they fill the lungs completely and make them expand. This activity helps the circulation of the blood in the lungs.

Sometimes the body forms more carbon dioxide than usual, especially during vigorous exercises. More rapid breathing quickly removes that carbon dioxide.

The prime reason for breathing properly while exercising is to prevent injury. Then the particular exercise can be completed with ease. Breathing at the right moment takes the strain off the muscles.

A general rule to follow is the EE rule, which is "Exhale on the Effort." The exceptions to the EE rule are noted with the exercise.

Exercises for Warming Up

That which you think today becomes that which you are tomorrow.

2 Exercises for Warming Up

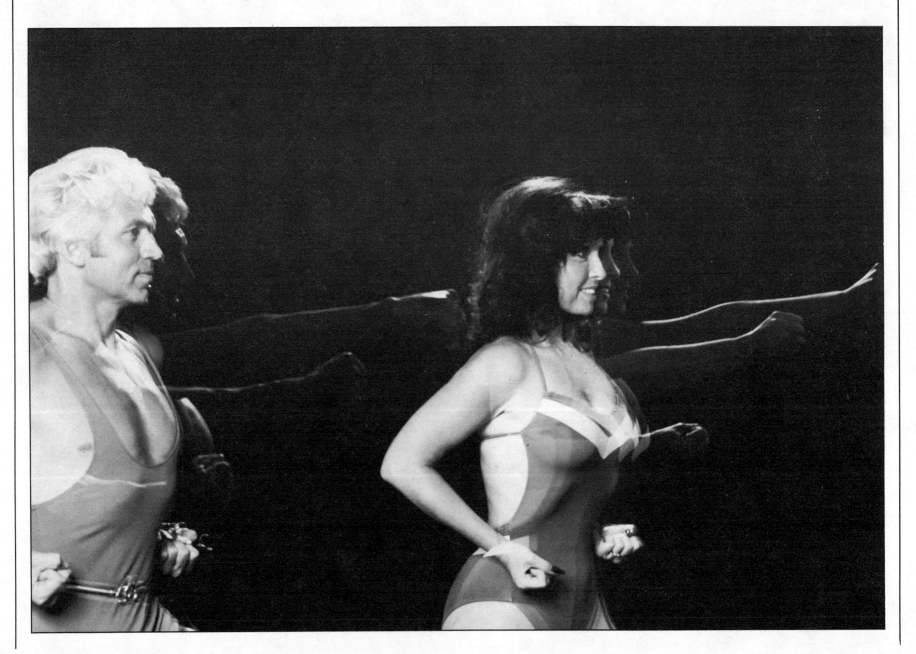

You're ready to start your exercise program. You've just purchased running shoes, shorts, T-shirts, a sweat suit. You already feel better about yourself. You can't wait to begin. Hold it. Slow down. Realize that nobody performs well without sufficient warm-up. Watch athletes an hour before a big game. Watch dancers backstage before a ballet. Watch musicians before a concert. They limber their joints, stretch muscles, prepare themselves for the more rigorous activity of the event. The same goes for you. You warm up in order to do the more strenuous exercises without damaging your muscles. So take it easy. Slowly stretch, lean, twist, reach. Enjoy the sensation as your muscles loosen up and come alive.

WARMING UP

Karate Lunge
Stand with your legs shoulder width apart, slightly bend knees. Punch with right fist while lunging forward with left knee. Return to starting position and repeat on other side. Inhale at the beginning, exhale on punch and lunge. Beginners should do 10 repetitions, work up to 50 reps as you become stronger.

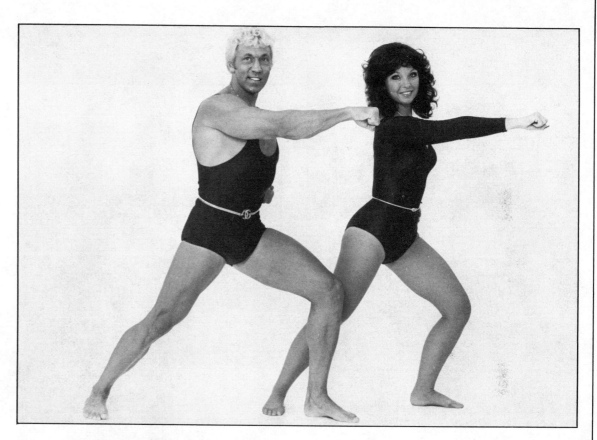

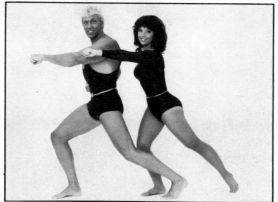

2 Exercises for Warming Up

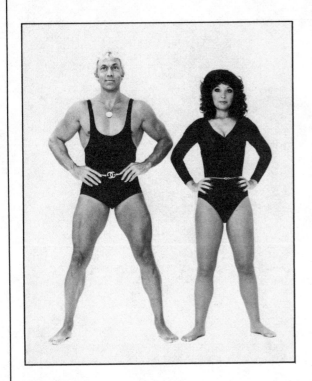

Stretches

Stand with legs apart, bend your knees, and tighten buttocks. Reach for ceiling with right arm, left arm is at your side. Then reach up with left arm while dropping right arm. Do this movement in 4 counts. Try this series of stretches for 4 sets. Inhale at start and exhale on stretch.

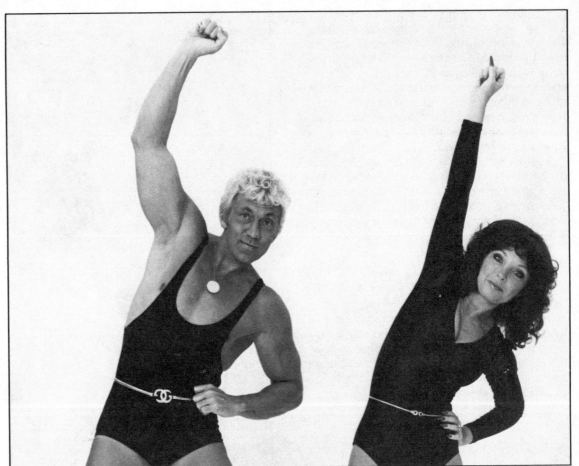

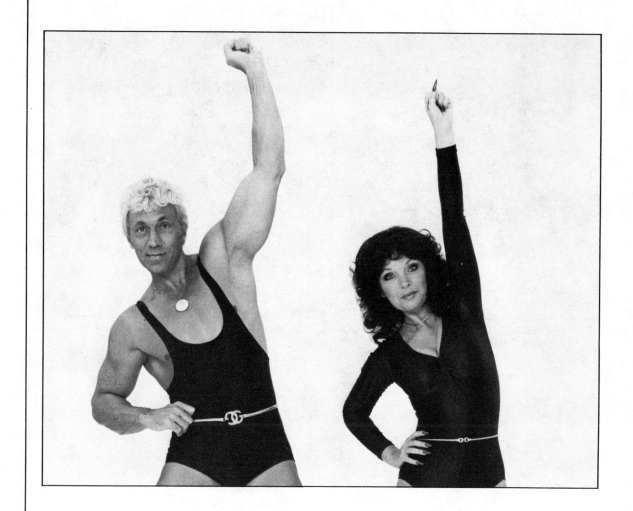

2 Exercises for Warming Up

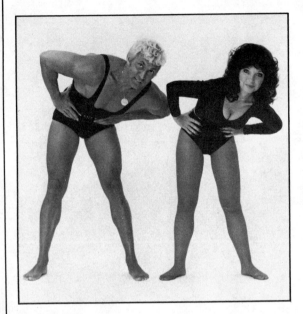
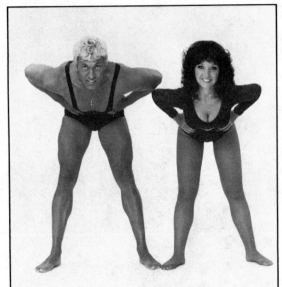
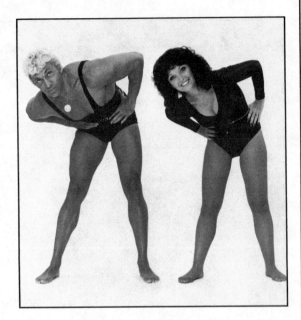

Body Bow Swing
Stand with legs apart, bend knees, and tighten
buttocks. Bend over at the waist, swing torso
to the left, then swing torso to the right (as a
pendulum swings). Inhale at center and exhale
at each side. Beginners do 10 reps, work up to
20 reps a day.

Puff, Pant, and Perspire

"Habit is a cable: We weave a thread of it every day, and at last we cannot break it."
Horace Mann

③ Puff, Pant, and Perspire

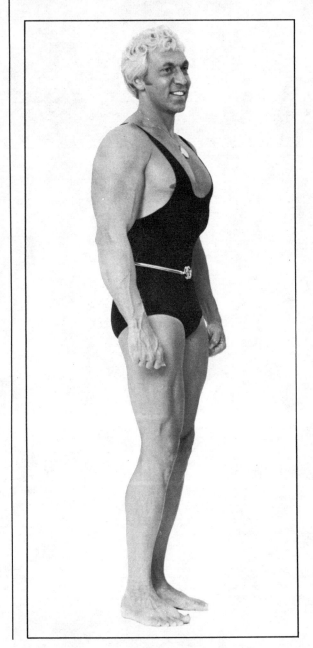

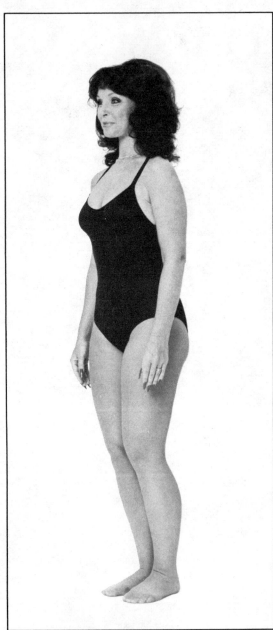

"I'm tired." "I'm bored." "I don't feel like I have any energy." These are frequent complaints from inactive men and women, most of whom are listless and have no stamina. These cardiovascular exercises get the old heart pumping, get the lungs expanding and contracting, and put a hefty supply of oxygen into the bloodstream. The increased stimulation to the heart and lungs produces beneficial changes in the body, resulting in increased endurance and healthier circulation. Physical fitness experts agree that the best medicine against heart disease is a strong cardiovascular system coupled with proper nutrition.

While doing these exercises it is important that you breathe properly. Inhale through the nose, exhale through the mouth. The rhythm of your breathing should coincide with the rhythm of the exercise. It is a fluid, graceful process. Consider yourself a dynamic art form.

So let's get with it. Puff, pant, and perspire for a longer, more vigorous life.

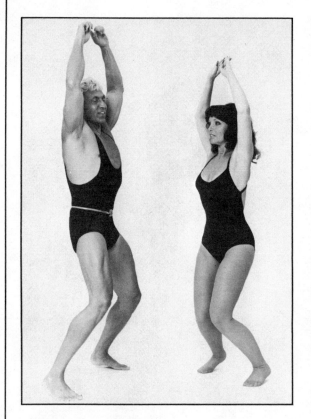

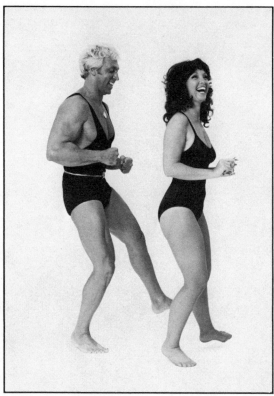

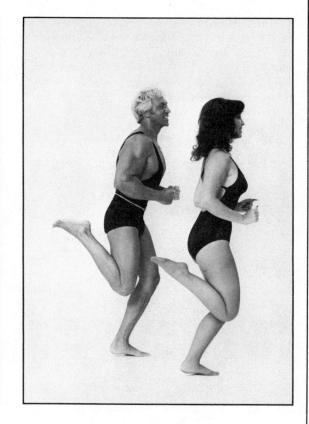

PUFF, PANT, PERSPIRE

Jumping Bodies (exercises cardiovascular-pulmonary system—heart, blood vessels, lungs)
Stand with feet together, unlock knees, put hands at sides, and inhale. Jump up, legs apart and raising hands overhead in one motion, exhale, and return to starting position. Beginners do 10 times, work up to 50 reps.

Dance Jog
Stand feet apart, hop and kick to either side one leg at a time. Breathe normally. Beginners should do 10 each side or a comfortable amount.

Kick Back (exercises back of thighs)
Stand feet together and kick back. Try to hit buttocks with heels, hopping from one leg to the other. Breathe normally. Beginners do 20 times or as many as you enjoy.

Puff, Pant, and Perspire

Fast Jog–Slow Jog

Fast Jog—try to bring knees to waist level for 10 counts. Breathe normally and jog in place, moving quickly. Slow Jog—barely move feet off floor while running in place for 10 counts. Breathe normally.

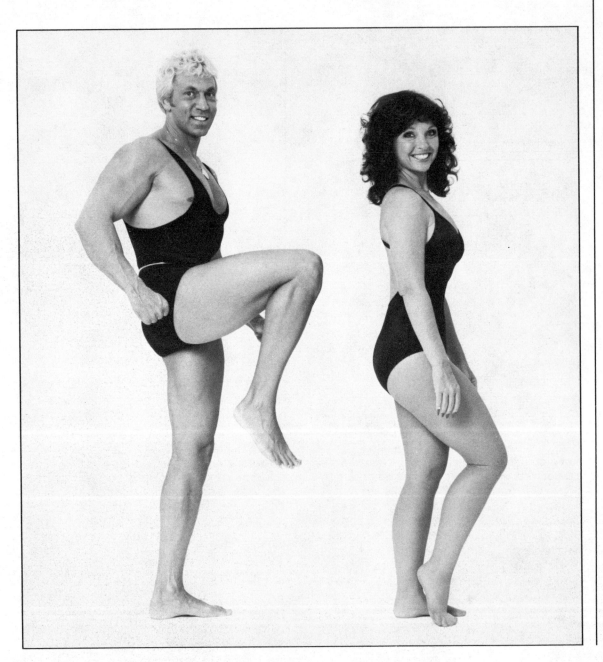

Success,

Bernie Ernst-

alendar

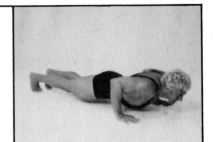

6 Do some light exercises today in addition to your Daily Dozens or job Now you are doing 10 reps per exercise of your Daily Dozens	**7** Today I exerplay* *Exerplay = exercise mixed with fun activities	**8** Starting weight this week _____ Do 15 reps of each exercise you choose in your Daily Dozens for the next six days	**9** I exercised today _____ Vary the exercises Do not strain your muscles	**10** I exercised today _____ At this point you will want to do more than advisable Have patience and proceed slowly
16 You are now half-way there—the worst is over You're on your way	**17** Remember you should be consistent in everything you do	**18** You are discouraged with your weight, but you will notice a change in the fit of your clothes	**19** Are your clothes much looser today? Yes _____ No _____ (If the answer is no, you are skipping days)	**20** Treat yourself— you deserve it Weight is important, but what you look like is more important Are you looking good?
26 HOORAY! You're practically there Don't stop now	**27** You are reaching pay dirt. Good exercise habits are being established	**28** Strictly fun day Enjoy. Look in your mirror	**29** Your new weight _____ Compare with first day _____ Positive proof the program works for you Take monthly measurements Chest _____ Waist _____ Hips _____ Thighs _____	**30** ★ I MADE IT.

ub. Send the tab at the
ll send you a free Body
/e will also send a new

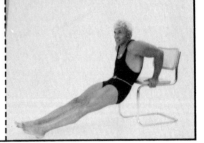

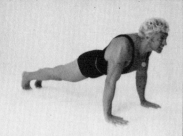

1 Starting weight _____ Start exercise program Start reducing program See nutrition chapter Start Daily Dozens for men Do 5 reps each exercise Measurements: Chest _____ Waist _____ Hips _____ Thighs _____	**2** Check I exercised today _____ I stayed on my reducing program _____ Add 1 rep to each exercise in your Daily Dozens How do I feel today? Write feeling _____	**3** Check I exercised today _____ I stayed on my reducing program _____ Drink Perrier Water (or some other water substitute) with lime instead of diet colas	**4** Do not stray Exercise today	**5** I exercised today _____ Do you feel badly today? Great, the program is working. Drink lots of water, it will get better
11 I exercised today _____ Your personal goals are important to be aware of	**12** I exercised today _____ After the routine today, the next two days are a snap	**13** Today I exercise Tomorrow I play Tonight—take a break Enjoy your dinner, eat healthy. Eat what you like	**14** Today we're back on our reducing program. Did you have a good time last night? Today I Exerplay	**15** Starting weight this week _____ Now you are doing 20 reps per exercise this week Don't give up. This is a tough period
21 Exerplay day Are friends beginning to notice a change?	**22** Starting weight this week _____ Now do 25 reps per exercise this week	**23** Energy will now start to surge for the new you to emerge	**24** Continue the 25 reps for each exercise	**25** Full steam ahead

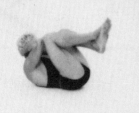

Now change your Daily Dozens for variety.
Choose your own Daily Dozens
from exercises in this book
Keep up the good work. We're with you.

You have now become a member of the "I Made It" Body Buddies c.
right to Nutrition Educators with your name and address and we w
Buddies T-shirt with your "I Made It" star emblazoned on the shirt.
30-day calendar free upon request. Check the boxes on the tab.

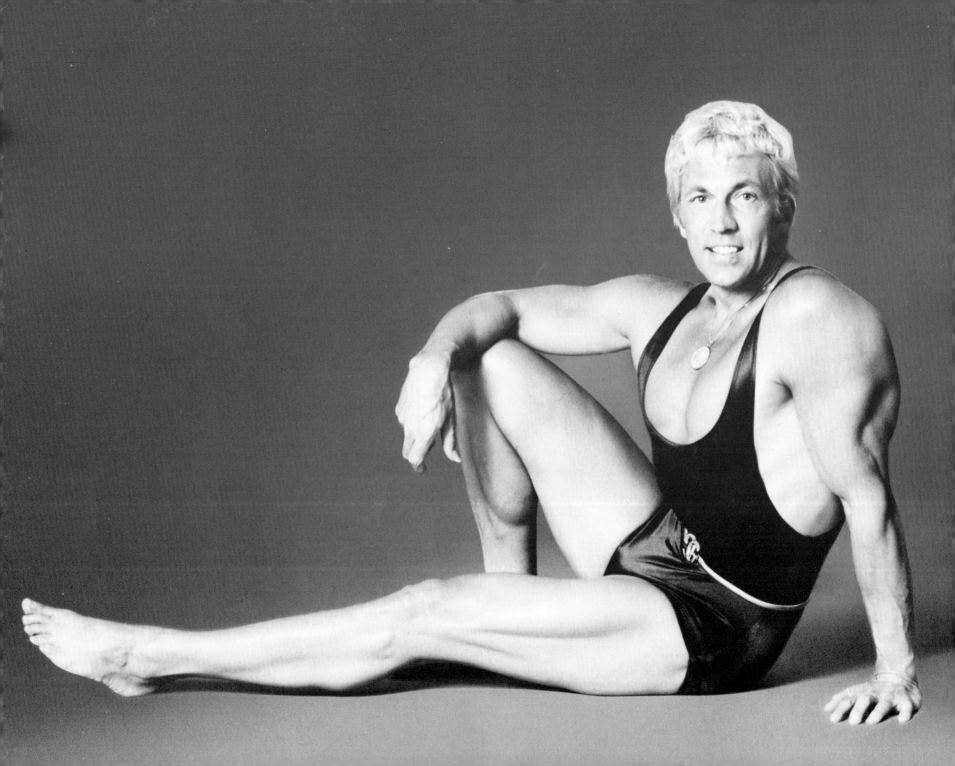

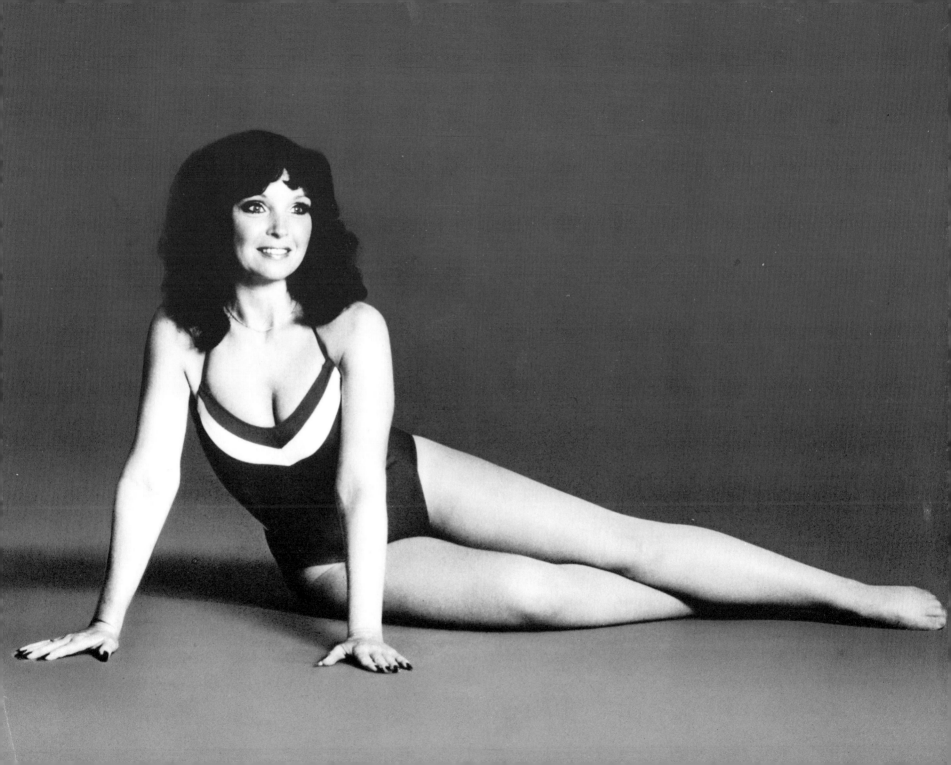

Calendar

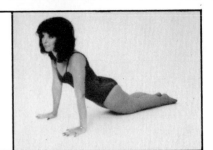

	7 Today I exerplay* *Exerplay = exercise mixed with fun activities	**8** Starting weight this week _____ Do 15 reps of each exercise you choose in your Daily Dozens for the next six days	**9** I exercised today _____ Vary the exercises Do not strain your muscles	**10** I exercised today _____ At this point you will want to do more than advisable Have patience and proceed slowly
o some light exercises day in addition to your aily Dozens or job ow you are doing reps per exercise your Daily Dozens				
ou are now half- ay there—the orst is over ou're on your way	**17** Remember you should be consistent in everything you do	**18** You are discouraged with your weight, but you will notice a change in the fit of your clothes	**19** Are your clothes much looser today? Yes _____ No _____ (If the answer is no, you are skipping days)	**20** Treat yourself— you deserve it Weight is important, but what you look like is more important Are you looking good?
OORAY! ou're practically there Don't stop now	**27** You are reaching pay dirt. Good exercise habits are being established	**28** Strictly fun day Enjoy. Look in your mirror	**29** Your new weight _____ Compare with first day _____ Positive proof the program works for you Take monthly measurements Bust _____ Waist _____ Hips _____ Thighs _____	**30** I MADE IT.

Send the tab at the
d you a free Body
ll also send a new

Mail this tab to the address below to receive your
new, free 30-day calendar and free Body Buddies T-shirt.

Mail to:
I MADE IT
Nutrition Educators
17932 Sky Park Blvd.
Irvine, Calif., 92714
Suite G
1-(714) 754-6414

Your phone no. (_____) _____ - _____
Name _____
Address _____
City _____
State _____ ZIP _____
Calendar ☐   T-shirt ☐

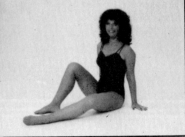

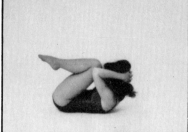

1
Starting weight _____
Start exercise program
Start reducing program
See nutrition chapter
Start Daily Dozens for women
Do 5 reps each exercise
Measurements:

Bust _____   Waist _____
Hips _____   Thighs _____

2   Check
I exercised today _____
I stayed on my
reducing program _____
Add 1 rep to each exercise
in your Daily Dozens
How do I feel today?
Write feeling _____

3   Check
I exercised today _____
I stayed on my
reducing program _____
Drink Perrier Water
(or some other water substitute)
with lime instead of diet colas

4
Do not stray
Exercise today

5
I exercised today _____
Do you feel badly today?
Great, the program
is working. Drink lots
of water, it will get better

11
I exercised today _____
Your personal goals
are important to
be aware of

12
I exercised today _____
After the routine
today, the next
two days are a snap

13
Today I exercise
Tomorrow I play
Tonight—take a break
Enjoy your dinner, eat
healthy. Eat what you like

14
Today we're back on our
reducing program. Did
you have a good time
last night?
Today I Exerplay

15
Starting weight
this week _____
Now you are doing
20 reps per exercise
this week
Don't give up. This is
a tough period

21
Exerplay day
Are friends beginning
to notice a change?

22
Starting weight
this week _____
Now do 25 reps per
exercise this week

23
Energy will now
start to surge
for the new you
to emerge

24
Continue the 25 reps
for each exercise

25
Full steam ahead

Change your Daily Dozens for variety. Choose your own
Daily Dozens from exercises in this book. Women may
experience weight gain because of their menstrual cycle,
but don't worry, it will go away.

You have now become a member of the "I Made It" Body Buddies club.
right to Nutrition Educators with your name and address and we will se
Buddies T-shirt with your "I Made It" star emblazoned on the shirt. We w
30-day calendar free upon request. Check the boxes on the tab.

Happiness,

Jeanne Ernst

Exercises for the Bustline, Chest, and Arms

Dieters: When you come to the end of your rope, tie a knot in it and hang on. Take a day off but don't give up—hang in there.

4 Exercises for the Bustline, Chest, and Arms

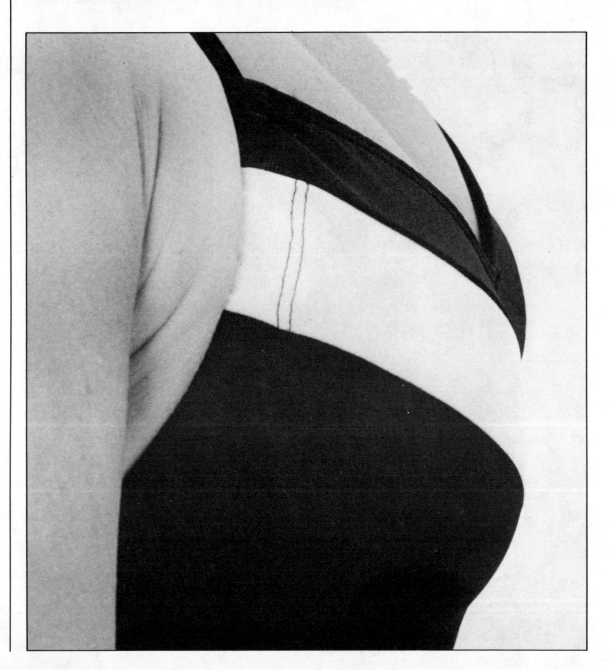

You're special. Your body has its own shape, its own form. You want to do the best with what you have—lose the excess weight, firm up the sagging muscles.

For years women have been inundated with an avalanche of methods and promises for larger breasts. Clever entrepreneurs, capitalizing on women's insecurities, have made millions of dollars on an array of gadgets that falsely claim to make the bustline bigger. In Hollywood, actresses enter hospitals for plastic surgery and silicone injections. We believe these methods to be somewhat drastic. The point is to go with what you've got, firming and developing muscles that already exist. All of us should do what we can do with what we have and make our bodies the best they can be. A muscle in its flabby state is loose and just hangs. When a woman starts training with resistance exercises (i.e., weights), she starts rebuilding muscle fiber and burning off fat. The muscle compresses, gets heavier, providing "shape"—even for flat-chested women.

Men have become soft and flabby. Their once hard muscles have lost strength and tone and are covered with fat. Fat is simply stored energy, the result of calories and carbohydrates that have not been burned off in activity. To trim fat and restore tone and strength to muscles you must combine physical activity and proper diet. Eat fewer calories and carbohydrates and exercise more.

Remember, weight loss alone won't put you in shape. Exercise will firm up the muscles so that you look and feel better.

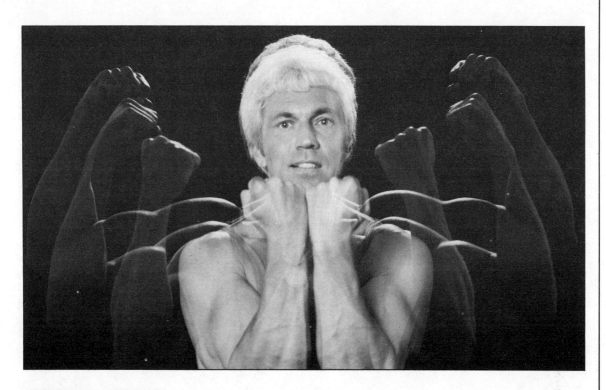

CHEST AND BUSTLINE

Firming Bustline (lifts and firms pectoral muscle)
Stand with legs apart, knees bent, bend elbows, tighten buttocks, and bring elbows back. Bring forearms and elbows together in front of you. Inhale with elbows back, exhale when forearms come together. Do 10 reps slowly, concentrate, and work up to 20 reps a day.

4 Exercises for the Bustline, Chest, and Arms

Push-Ups (exercises bustline for women and chest for men, back of arms, and shoulders)

● Women (beginners)
Start on hands and knees, palms flat, elbows straight. Slowly lower body to the floor by bending elbows. Do not touch the floor, then push up slowly by straightening elbows. Inhale going down, exhale as you push up.
Start with 10 reps, work up to 20 reps a day before advancing to full push-ups.

● Men (advanced)
Hands on floor, palms flat, back is flat, legs straight, toes touching floor. Inhale going down, exhale as you push up. Start with 10 reps, work up to 50 a day.

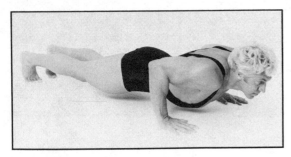

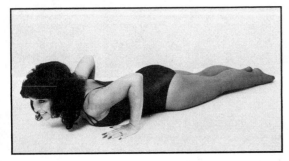

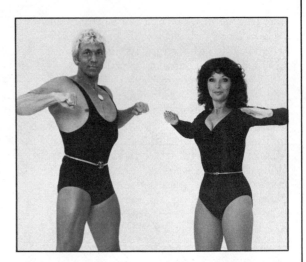

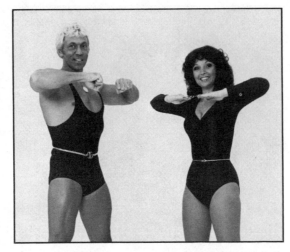

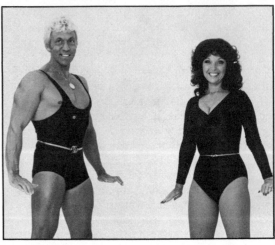

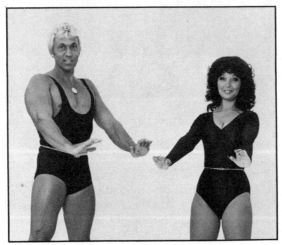

ARMS

Elbows Back-2 Down-2 (exercises posture, back muscles and back of arms)
Stand with legs apart, unlock or relax knees. Raise arms, elbows bent. Pull elbows back for 2 counts and inhale. Drop arms to side of body, extend wrists back for 2 counts and exhale. Do 10 reps, work up to 20 reps.

Reverse Hand Pushout Overhead (works back of arms and chest)

Stand with legs apart, unlock and relax knees. Clasp hands together, turn palms out. Place against chest for starting position. Push palms out—count 1, raise overhead—count 2, back—count 3, return to chest—count 4. Inhale at start. Exhale on 1, inhale on 2, exhale on 3, inhale on 4. Do 10 times, work up to 20 reps a day.

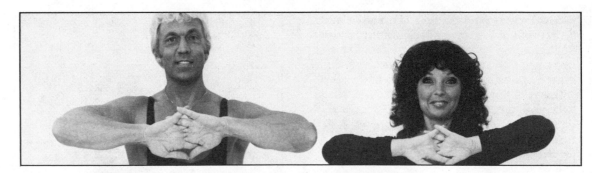

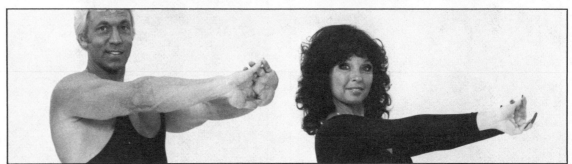

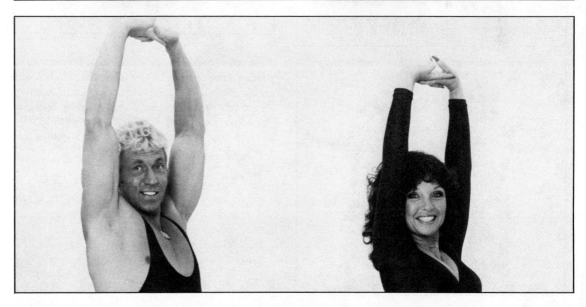

4 Exercises for the Bustline, Chest, and Arms

Elbow Twist (exercises back of arms—triceps)
Stand with legs apart, unlock or relax knees, tighten buttocks. Start with raised arms straight and out from sides at shoulder height, fist turned toward ceiling. Now rotate first backwards. Continue rotation until you feel tension in back of arm. Inhale starting position, exhale finished position. Do 10 times, work up to 20 reps a day.

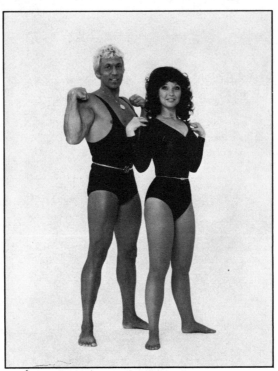

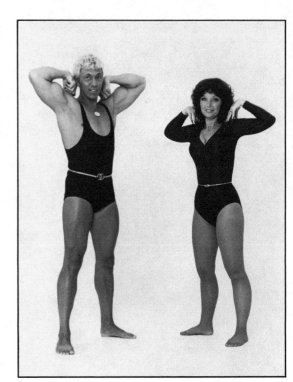

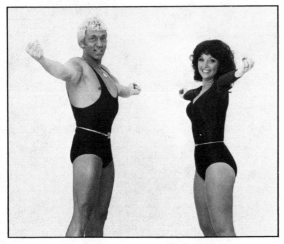

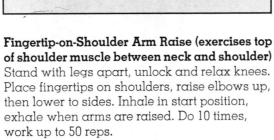

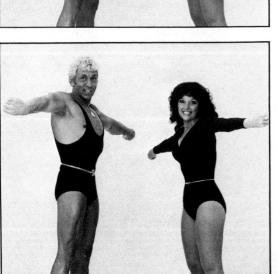

Fingertip-on-Shoulder Arm Raise (exercises top of shoulder muscle between neck and shoulder)
Stand with legs apart, unlock and relax knees. Place fingertips on shoulders, raise elbows up, then lower to sides. Inhale in start position, exhale when arms are raised. Do 10 times, work up to 50 reps.

Exercises for the Waist and Stomach

Anything that causes us to worry is not worth what worry costs us.

5 Exercises for the Waist and Stomach

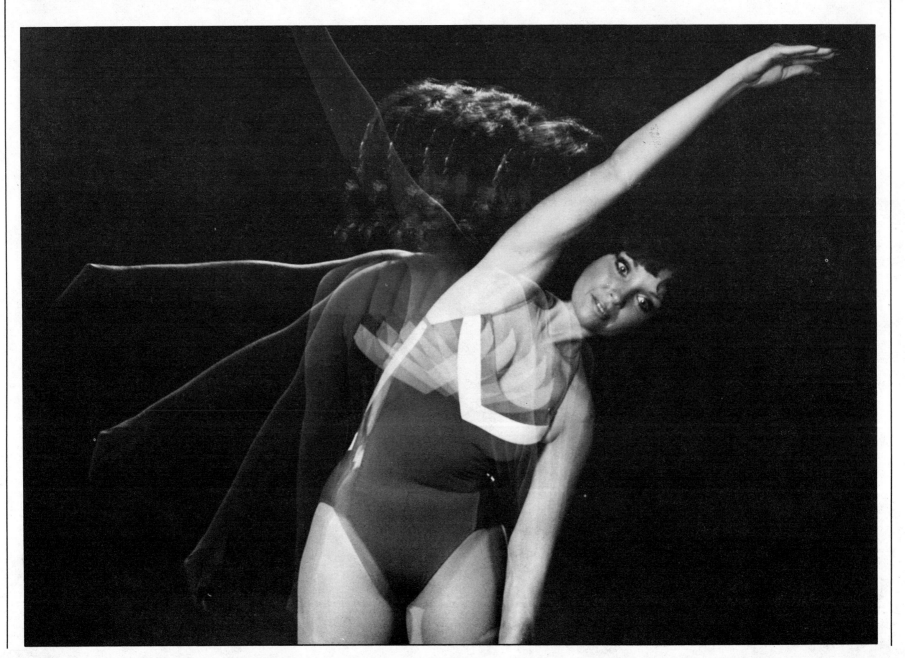

Years of irresponsible eating and drinking habits, along with a lack of physical activity, have created the unsightly stomach overhang that precedes us through every door. Lacking the personal discipline to do anything about our condition, we've accepted the humiliation associated with our pot bellies and unglamorous "love handles." Is the pleasure of eating and drinking worth the ugly flab we mask with gunny-sack dresses and suits that look like tents?

By following the Daily Dozens, or just the few exercises on the following pages, you will surprise yourself, and in just a short time watch the disappearance of all that fat. Remember, count your calories, too.

Carrying less weight diminishes the strain on your heart and provides you with renewed vigor reflected by a lighter step and a better attitude about yourself.

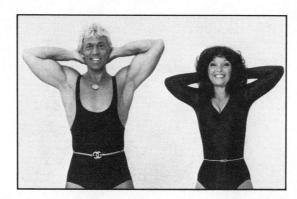
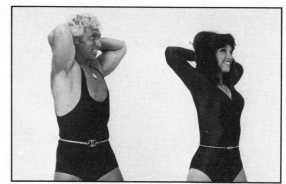

WAIST

Hands Behind Head Waist Twist (exercises entire waist)

Stand with legs apart, unlock knees. Place hands behind head. Twist from side to side. Inhale at center, exhale on twist. Beginners do 10 times, work up to 50 reps.

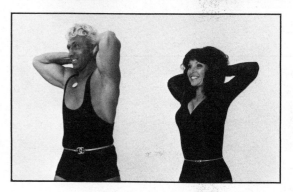

26

Extended Palm Side Reach (exercises side of waist)

Stand with legs apart, unlock knees. Extend wrist away from body. Inhale, bend over to the side, and exhale. Repeat on other side. Beginners do 10 on each side, work up to 50 reps a day, slowly.

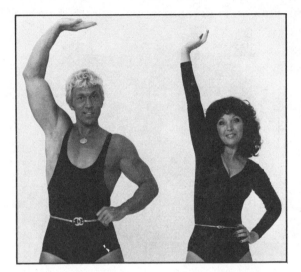
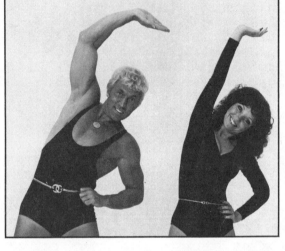
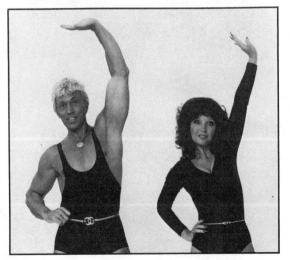
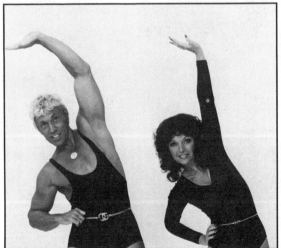

2-Count Press Arm Change (exercises chest, waist, back, and arms)

Stand with legs apart, unlock knees. Raise left arm straight in front of you. Right arm back and bent. Push-pull motion for 2 counts, then change to other side. Inhale and exhale each arm change. Beginners do 10 reps, work up to 20 reps.

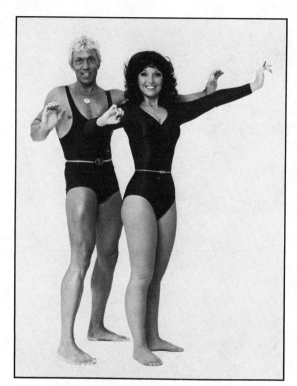

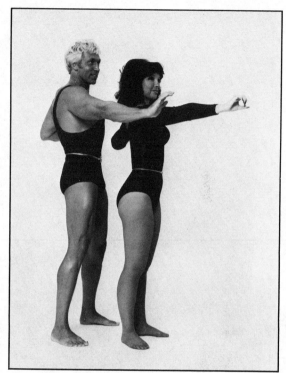

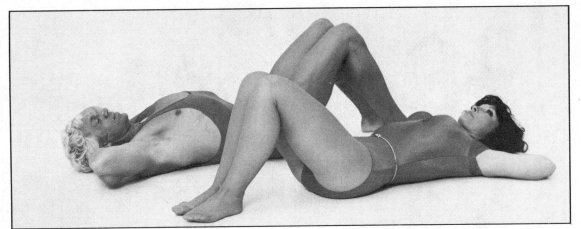

STOMACH

Crunch and Twist (exercises stomach and waist)

Lie on floor, hands behind head, bend knees, and inhale. Bring shoulders up off floor and twist side to side. Count 1, 2, 3, 4 and exhale. Return to floor and inhale. Beginners do 10 reps, work up to 20 reps.

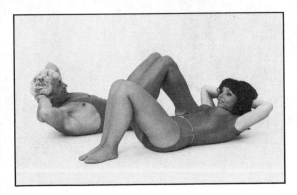

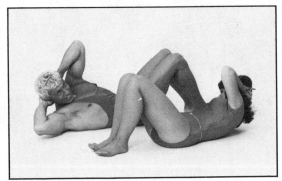

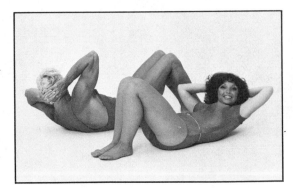

Single Knee Squeeze (exercises lower stomach and upper stomach)

Lie on floor, hands behind head, bend knees. Bring head and shoulders up off floor and squeeze one knee with elbows. Inhale on starting position, exhale on squeeze. Do 10 reps one side and repeat on other side, work up to 50 reps on each side.

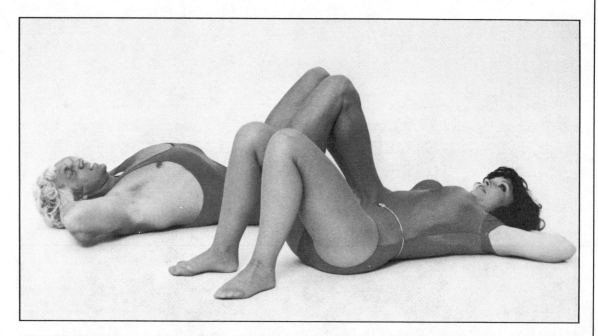

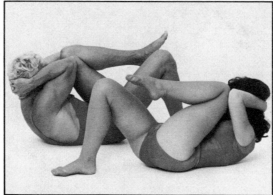

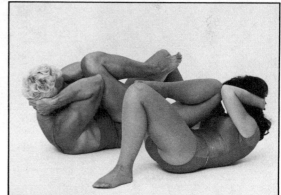

5 Exercises for the Waist and Stomach

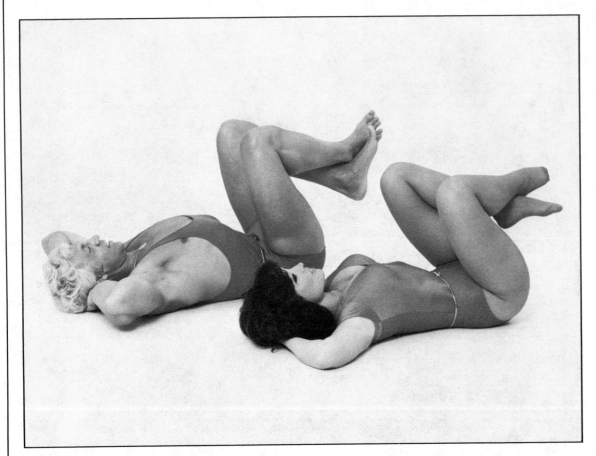

Quarter Sit-Up (exercises entire stomach)
Lie on floor, bend knees, hands behind head, and inhale. Now exhale, sit up, and touch elbows to knees. Do this exercise at a good pace and with a smooth rhythm. Always exhale on stomach squeeze. Beginners do 10, work up to 50 reps.

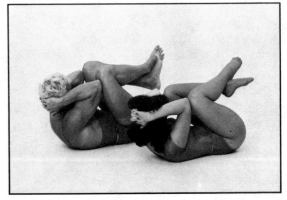

Ankle cross—elbow to knee (exercises stomach)
Lie on floor, hands behind head, cross ankles,
inhale, bring knees and elbows together and
touch elbow to opposite knee. Exhale and
return feet to floor and repeat on other side.
Beginners do 10 times, work up to 20 reps a
day.

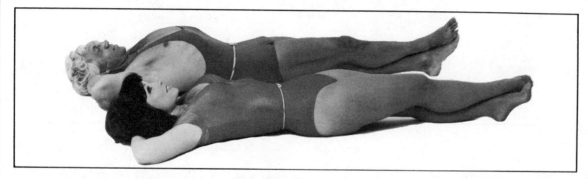

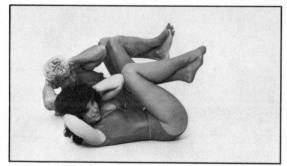

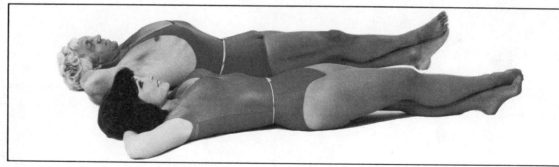

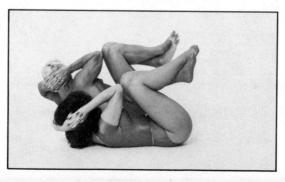

32 **Side Knee-Up—Straight Leg-Up (exercises hips, lower stomach, and thighs)**
Lie on left side, legs together and straight. Recline on left elbow—right hand in front or behind body for support. Inhale, bring knees up toward torso. Exhale, return legs to starting position. Repeat on other side. Beginners do 10 reps, work up to 20 reps.

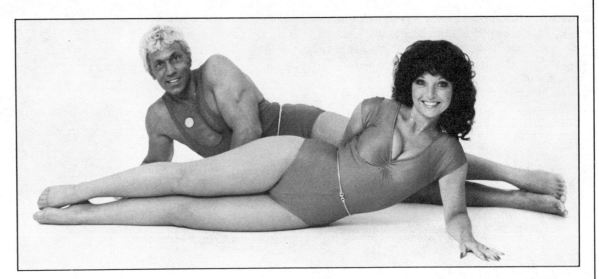

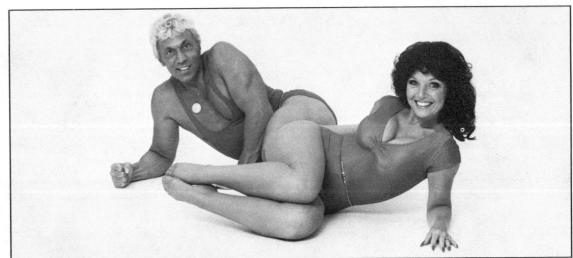

Exercises for the Buttocks, Hips, Thighs and Calves

"Do what you can, with what you have, where you are."
Teddy Roosevelt

6 Exercises for the Buttocks, Hips, Thighs and Calves

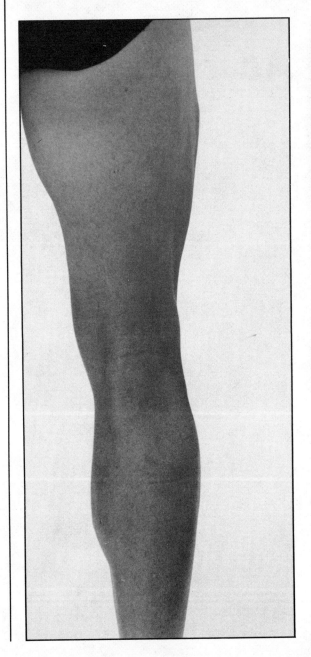

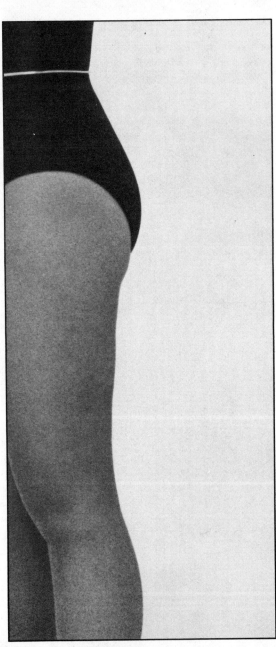

We give little thought to the buttocks and hips during the winter months, even less to the thighs and calves. However, as the weather warms and beaches and swimming pools beckon, these areas of our anatomy become more visible. Nothing turns off a man or woman more than seeing flabby buttocks oozing from a bathing suit. Fat and wrinkled thighs are equally unattractive. Women also feel repulsed when they see a nice-looking man with a fat posterior and pudgy, unmuscled legs.

Well, what are you waiting for? Shape those hips and thighs. Firm up your buttocks and calves. Get ready for that summer or winter vacation. You'll be glad you did.

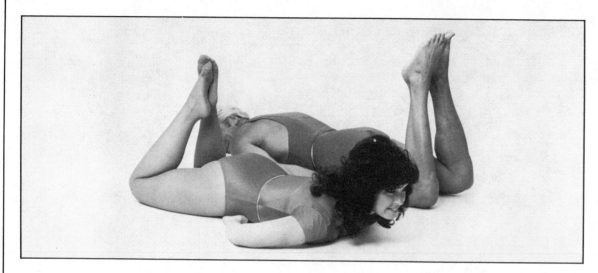

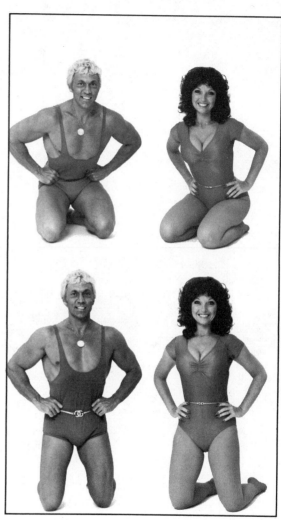

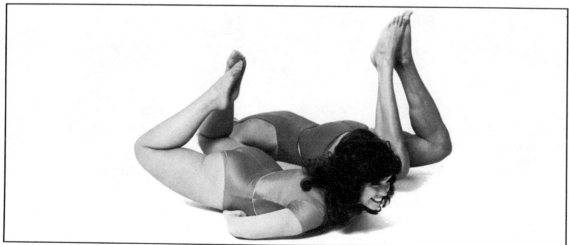

BUTTOCKS

Swim Thigh Slap (exercises inner thigh and buttocks)

Lie on stomach, place hands under pelvis (to protect lower back). Tighten buttocks and slap thighs together. Inhale at start, exhale on slap. Beginners do 10 reps, work up to 30 reps a day.

Kneeling Pelvic Tilt (exercises buttocks, hips, and thighs)

Kneel on a pillow or soft carpet, sit on heels, and inhale. Rise to kneeling position and squeeze buttocks together, then exhale. Do not arch back, keep body in a straight line. Beginners do 10 reps, work up to 50 reps a day.

6 Exercises for the Buttocks, Hips, Thighs and Calves

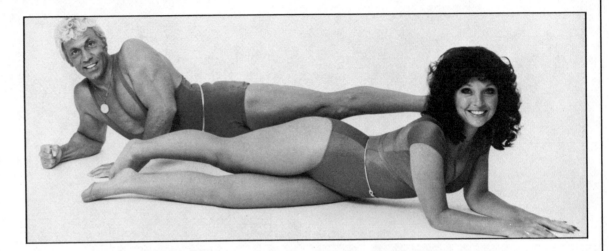

Extended Heel—Back Leg Lift (exercises buttocks)

Lie on your side, roll forward slightly, put toe on floor, heel pointed toward ceiling. Lift leg straight up, tighten buttocks. Inhale at starting position, exhale as leg is lifted. Beginners do 10 reps, then turn over and do other side. Work up to 50 reps a day.

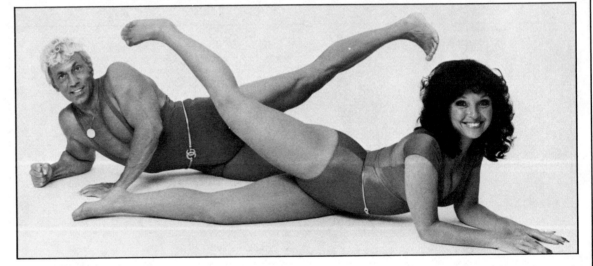

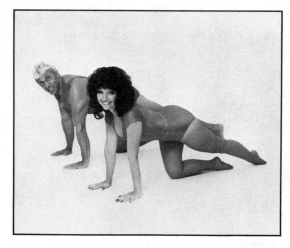

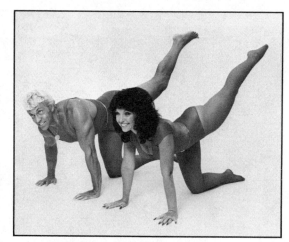

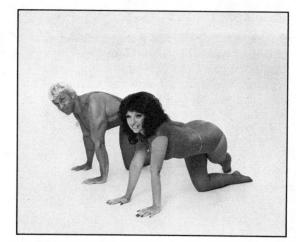

Donkey—4 Count Leg Lift (exercises buttocks)
Kneel. On hands and knees, palms flat, one leg straight back. Lift leg and inhale, cross over other leg and exhale. Lift leg up, inhale, return to floor, and exhale. Beginners do 10 reps, then repeat on other side. Work up to 20 reps each side.

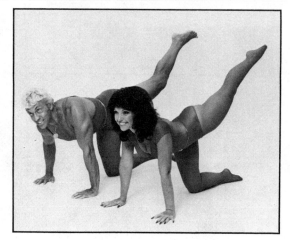

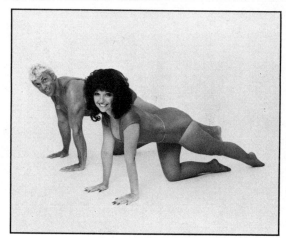

HIPS AND THIGHS

Donkey Kicks, Side and Back (exercises side of thigh, back of thigh, and buttocks.)
On hands and knees, lift knee to shoulder, and inhale. Kick to the side and exhale. Return knee to shoulder and inhale, kick back, and exhale. Beginners do 10 reps, then do other side. Work up to 20 reps per day.

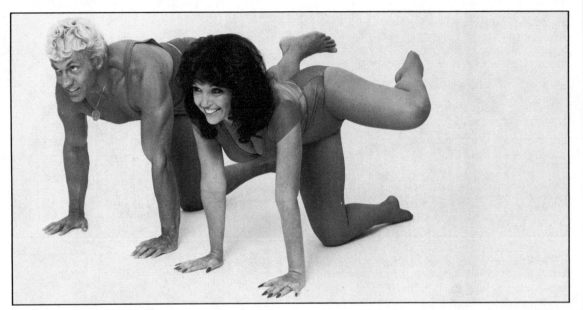

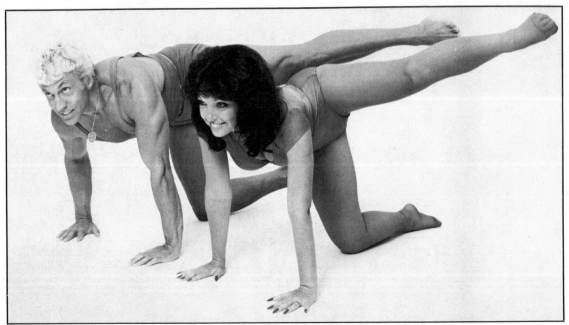

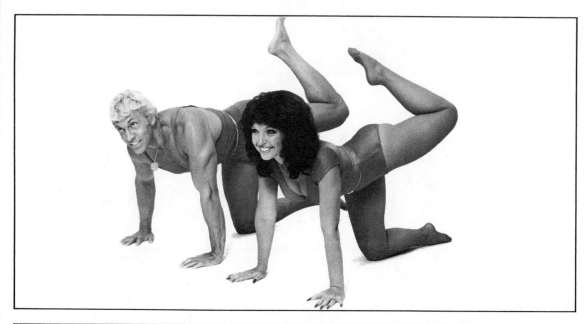

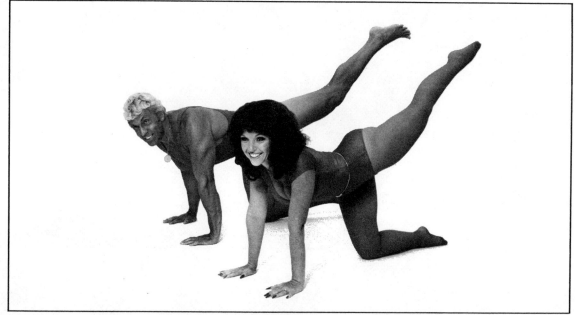

40

Hold Knee Leg Lift (exercises top of thigh)
Lie on back, hold one knee, other leg straight
on floor and inhale. Exhale as you raise leg.
Beginners do 10 reps, then repeat on other
side. Work up to 50 reps each side.

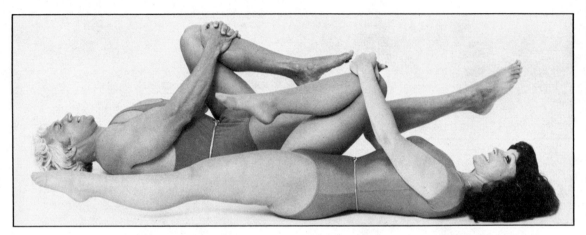

**Pivot Point Knee Bend (exercises hips and
entire thigh)**
Stand with legs apart, unlock knees, tighten
buttocks. Reach for an imaginary wall in front
of you with your hands and arms straight out
and reach for another wall with your bottom.
(Do not do a knee bend.) Return to starting
position. Inhale at starting position, exhale as
you reach forward. This exercise is excellent
for working hips and thighs without hurting
the lower back or placing stress on the knees.
Beginners do 10 reps, work up to 50 reps. For
picture see page 82.

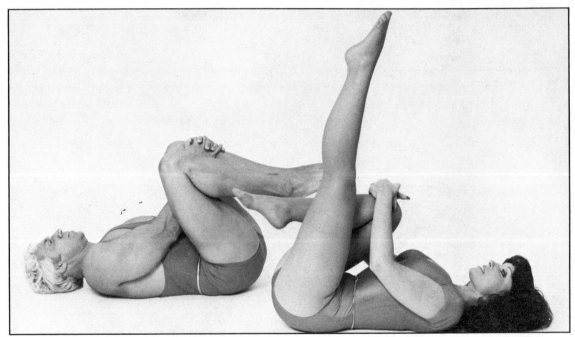

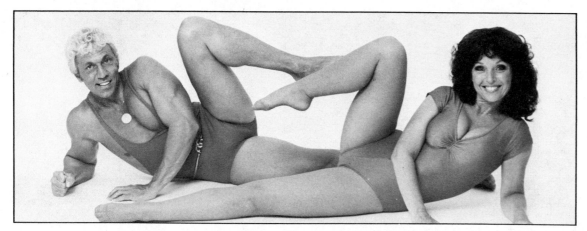

Side Knee-Up Straight Leg-Up (exercises hips and thighs)

Lie on left side, legs together and straight. Recline on left elbow, right hand in front of body for support. Inhale and bring knee up to shoulder, exhale, then straight back down and inhale, then back up to shoulder with straight leg and exhale. Repeat on other side. Do 10 reps on each side, work up to 20 reps.

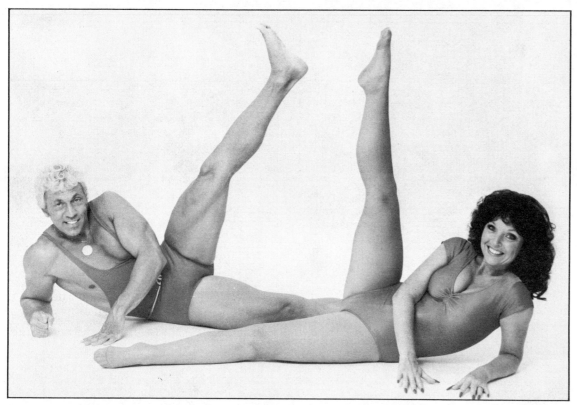

⑥ Exercises for the Buttocks, Hips, Thighs and Calves

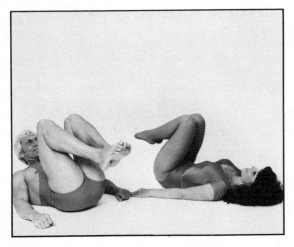

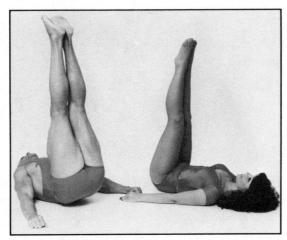

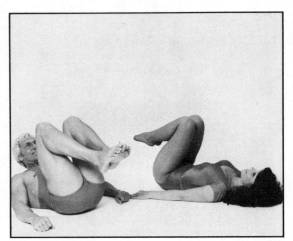

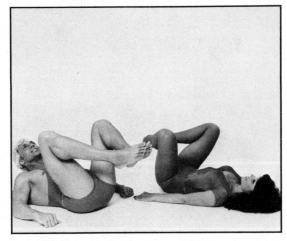

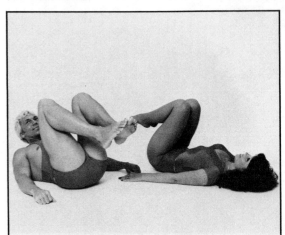

Up, Down, and Out Together (exercises top of thigh, side of thigh, and inner thigh)

Lie on your back and bend legs. Pull stomach in, bring knees to chest and inhale. Exhale as you straighten legs. Inhale as knees return to chest. Open knees and exhale. Slap knees together (not hard) and inhale. Beginners do 10 reps, work up to 50 reps.

One Leg Bounce (exercises top of thigh)
Sit on floor, bend one knee. Place hands around knee, keeping back straight. Pull stomach in, lift straight leg off floor, and bounce legs 5 times. Beginners do 5 reps, 10 for advanced. Change legs and repeat on other side. Breathe normally.

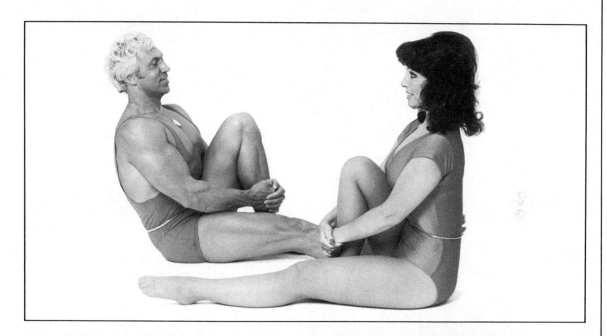

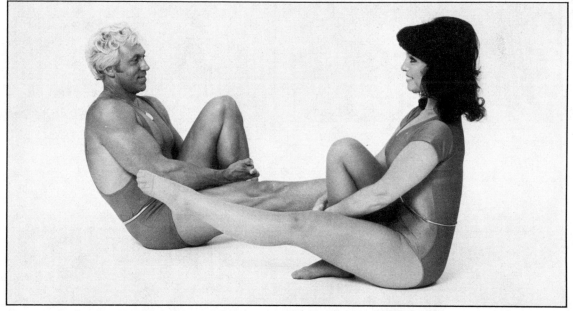

⑥ Exercises for the Buttocks, Hips, Thighs and Calves

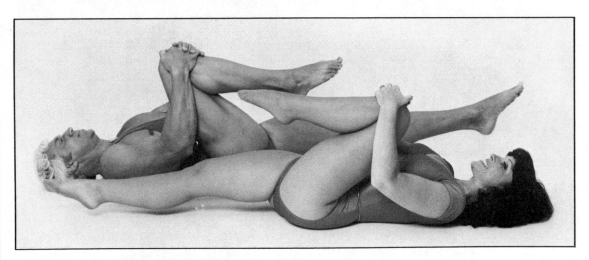

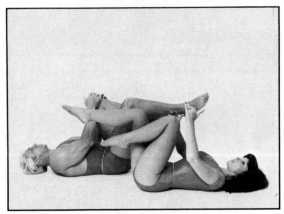

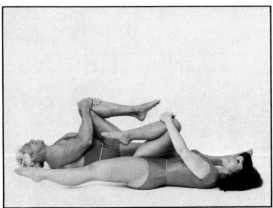

Hold Knee 2-Count Leg Change (exercises top of thigh and protects low back)

Lie on floor, pull stomach in, hold one knee, and inhale. Pull toward chest for 2 counts, and exhale. Change legs. Beginners do 10 times, work up to 20 reps per day.

INNER THIGH

Weighted Inner Thigh (exercises inner thigh)
Lie on side with legs straight, bend top knee,
and inhale. Lift bottom leg up and exhale. The
weight of the top leg is the resistance. Beginners do 10 reps, work up to 20 reps.

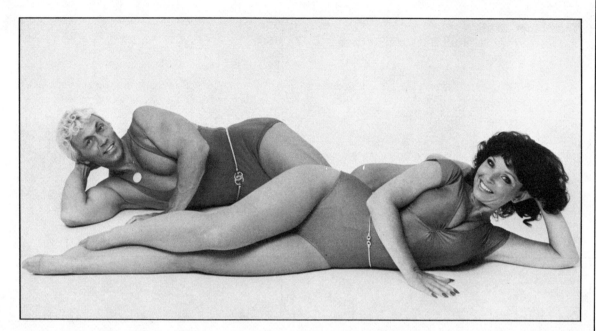

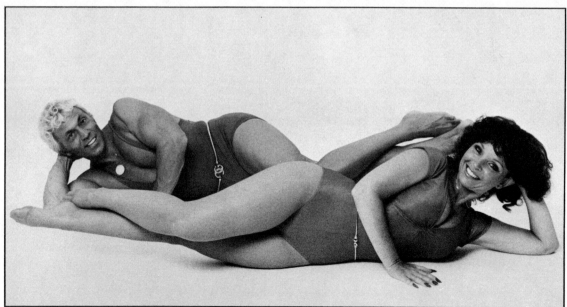

46

Lazy Inner Thigh

Lie on side with legs straight, support head with hand. Rest top leg on floor in front of bottom leg. Inhale, lift bottom leg off floor as high as possible, exhale on lift. Do as many as possible without straining. Repeat on other side.

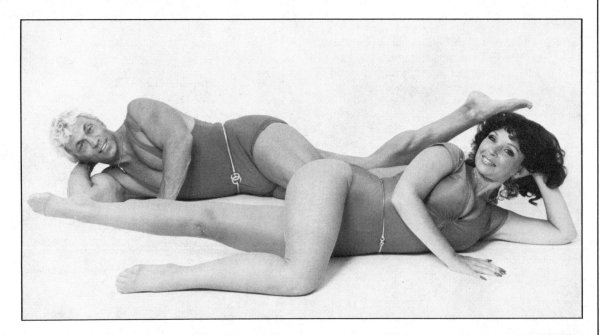

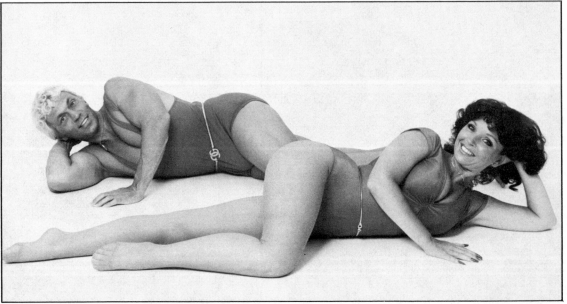

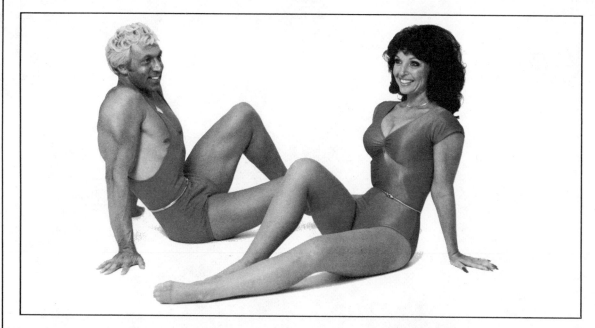

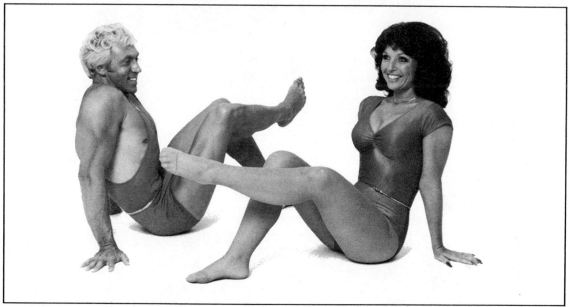

Inner Thigh Slice

Sit on the floor, pull stomach in, bend one knee. The other leg is slightly bent on the floor with knee turned out. Inhale, lift the leg in a slicing motion up to bent knee while exhaling. Return leg to floor and repeat. Beginners do 10 reps on each side, work up to 20 reps per side.

47

BACK OF THIGH

Donkey Leg Curl (exercises back of thigh and buttock)

On hands and knees, raise one leg straight out behind you. Now curl foot toward buttocks and exhale. Return to starting position and repeat. Beginners do 10 reps each side, work up to 50.

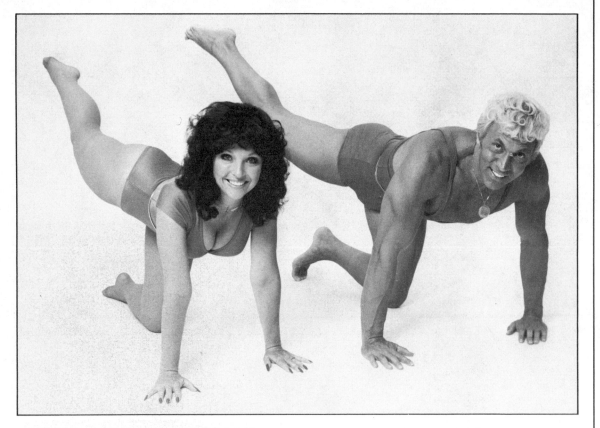

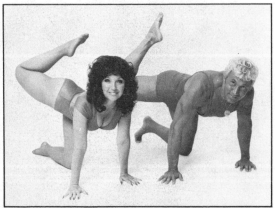

Beginners Leg Curls (exercises back of thigh)
Lie on stomach, hands under chin, legs
straight. Inhale, curl feet to buttocks, exhale.
Return to starting position and repeat. Beginners do 20 reps, work up to 50 reps per side.

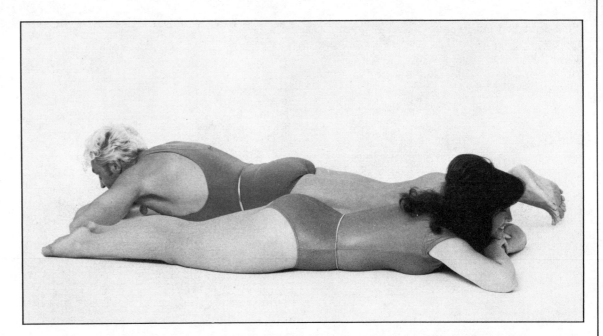

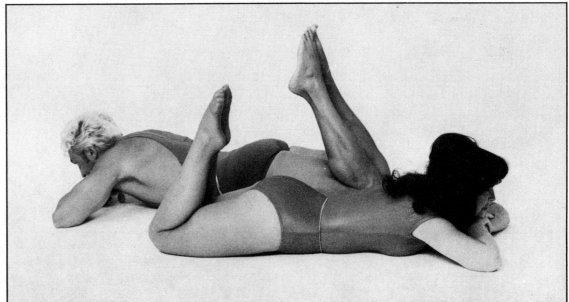

6 Exercises for the Buttocks, Hips, Thighs and Calves

Side Back Leg Lift (exercises back of thigh)
Lie on your side with legs straight and inhale.
Lift top leg to the back and up, tighten buttock
and exhale. Do 10 reps each leg, work up to
20 reps per side.

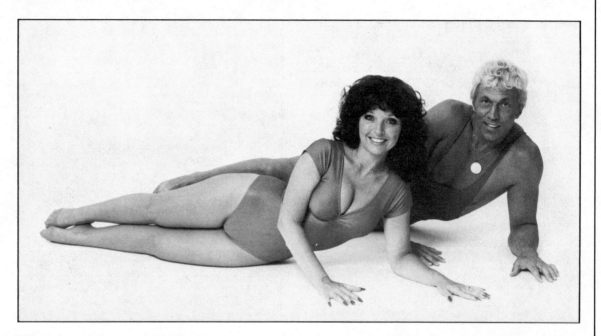

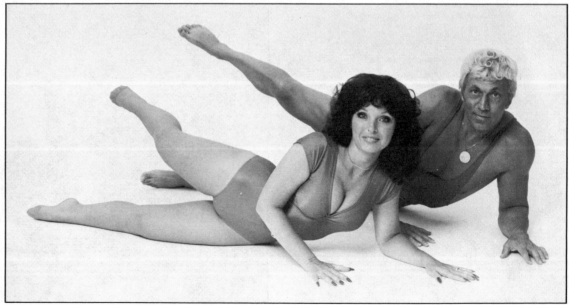

CALVES

Toe Raise

Stand with feet apart (beginners hold on to a chair for balance) and inhale, rise up on toes and exhale, and return heels to floor. Beginners do 10 reps, work up to as many as you can do.

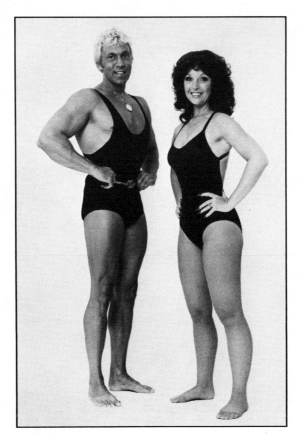

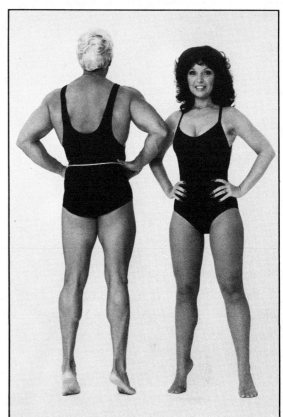

52

Toe Press (beginners)

Sit on the floor with legs straight. Pull stomach in, point toes to ceiling. Point toes forward. Beginners do 20 reps, work up to as many as you enjoy.

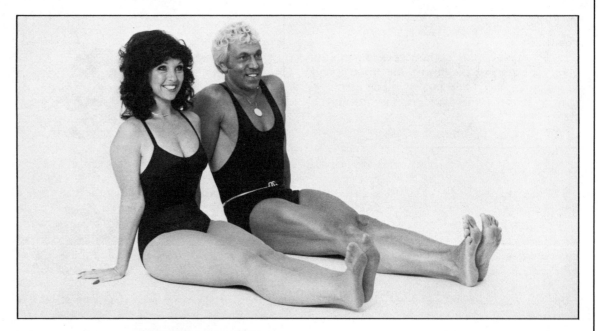

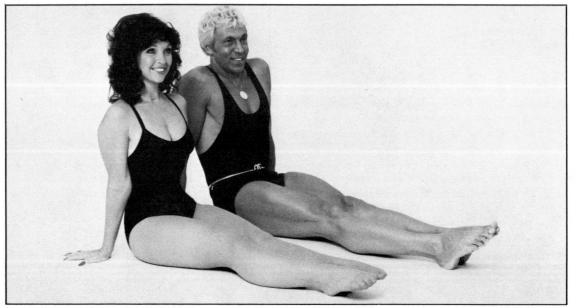

Exercises for the Lower Back

Those who do the most, dream the most.

7 Exercises for the Lower Back

The lower back is one of the weakest, most abused parts of our body. It needs to be stretched and twisted in order to strengthen and develop the muscles. It is wise to visit a chiropractor or physician before starting any strenuous back exercises.

Try to do a wide straddle toe touch. Be sure to bend your knees before attempting the exercise. Repeat once or twice, tightening the buttocks each time. Pretty soon you'll find you can put your palms flat on the floor. Also, waist twists with hands behind your head are good for initially limbering the back muscles. Remember, warm up gradually.

Do not move in a manner contrary to the natural inclination of your body. Trying to arch your back in an uncomfortable direction will be the cause of many aches and pains.

The lower back carries most of the burden for secretaries, engineers, telephone operators, artists, shoe salesmen—people whose occupations require that they sit or stand in bent-over positions for long periods of time. It is important for them to take an exercise break every once in a while to alleviate the stress and tension in the lower back. We believe that businesses would function more efficiently if instead of coffee breaks employees would take an exercise break.

Move, stretch, stand up, twist in your chair, pull your shoulders back a few times, and forget how you think you may look to others. Get a "body buddy." Ask a fellow worker to join you in your exercises. Your colleagues may learn something from your example.

Exercise is not a dirty word!

LOW BACK EXERCISES

These exercises are designed to strengthen the lower back and stretch the lower back muscles.

Hold Knee Leg Swing

Lie on your back, bring one knee up to chest and hold. Inhale, swing straight leg up and over while exhaling. Return to starting position. Do 10 swings on each side.

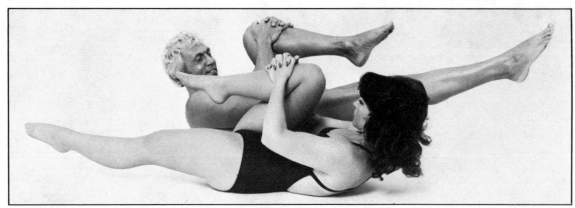

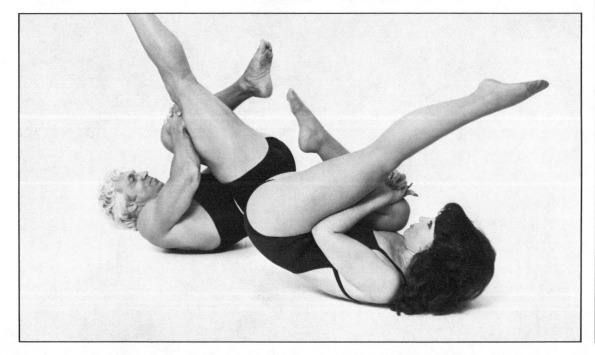

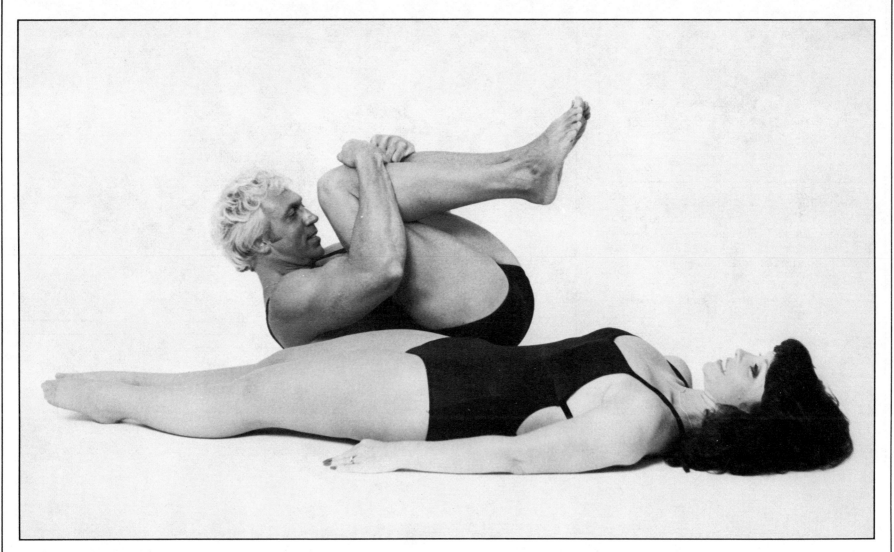

Double Knee Leg Pull

Lie on your back with legs straight and inhale. Slowly pull both knees up to chest while exhaling. Hug knees to chest for 4 counts. Return to starting position slowly. Do 10 times or as many as comfortable.

Single Knee Leg Pull

Same as double knee leg pull but use one knee at a time and keep opposite leg on the floor.

1 Exercises for the Lower Back

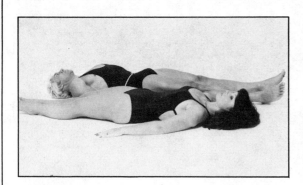

Spine on Floor
Lie on the floor, legs straight, inhale deeply. Slightly arch back. Put spine on the floor while tightening stomach muscles and exhale slightly, bending knees. Do as many as you enjoy.

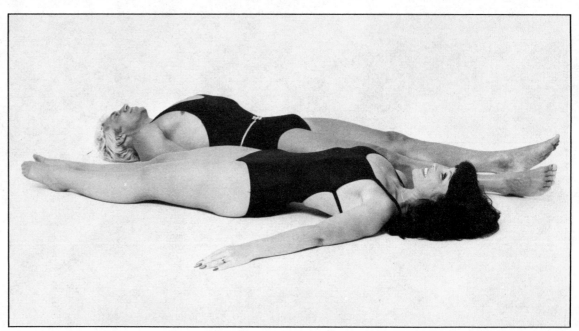

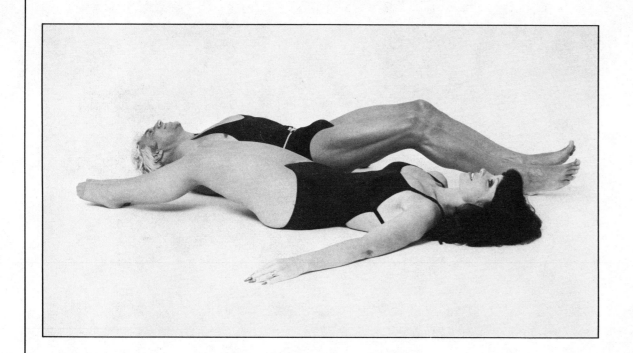

58

Cat Stretch

Put hands and knees on the floor, inhale and arch back with head up, then exhale. Pull stomach up and in, and exhale. Do as many as comfortable.

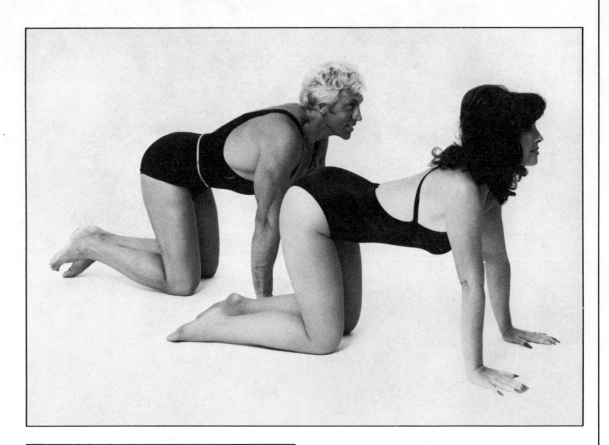

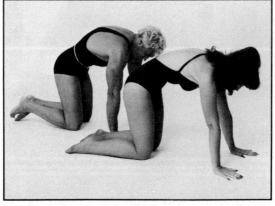

Jogging Warm-Ups

🎱 Jogging Warm-Ups

STRETCHES FOR WARMING UP

Stretching Pelvic Tilt (stretches top of thigh and exercises buttocks)
Knees on floor, arms straight, hands on floor behind you, buttocks resting on heels. Inhale and lift pelvis forward. Tighten buttocks and exhale, return to heels. Do 5 times.

Sprinters Stretch (stretches back of thigh, back of calf, and Achilles tendon)
Hands flat on floor, bend knees, buttocks on heels. Move one leg back, front leg bent, leg straight, heel on floor, slowly stretch. Hold for 10 counts, move leg forward, and put chest on thigh, for advanced. For beginners, stretch as far as comfortable. Hold for 10 counts. Do 4 with each leg, breathe normally.

Cross Ankle Toe Touch (stretches back of thigh)
Standing, cross right foot over left, bend forward, legs straight but don't strain, and touch floor. (Beginners stretch as far as possible.) Stop if muscles hurt. Hold for 10 to 30 seconds, then rise. Cross left foot over right and repeat forward bend. Do 5 times in each position.

Hold Ankle Windmill (stretches back of thigh)
Stand with legs apart, place left hand on right ankle (beginners hold calf), right arm straight out. Hold for 10 to 30 seconds. Then rise and put right hand on left ankle or calf, hold and stretch. Breathe normally. Do 5 times.

Seated Hamstring Stretch
Sit on the floor, pull stomach in, point toes to ceiling, put hands on toes and pull heels off floor. (Beginners hold calves in place of toes and stretch). Hold for 10 to 30 seconds. Breathe normally. Do 5 times.

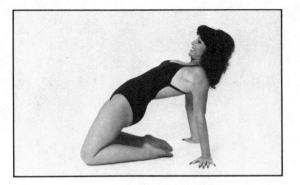

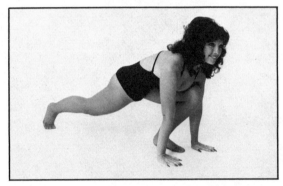

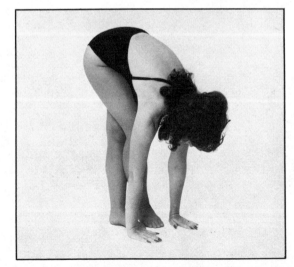

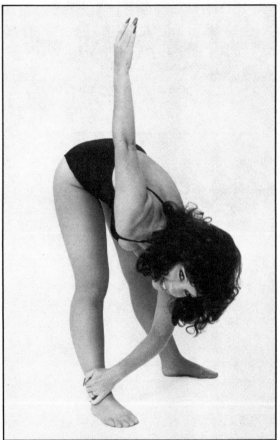

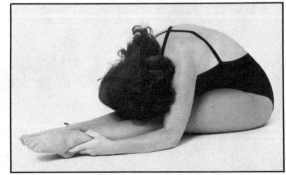

JOGGING

A MARATHON IN THE WORKS

The grueling twenty-six-mile marathon event has become a symbol of physical fitness in cities throughout the United States. Each year the number of participants increases by the thousands. Jogging has almost become our national pastime. When that five o'clock whistle blows, executives, secretaries, and laborers don their sweatsuits and running shoes and head for their favorite beaches, parks, and streets to get in their miles.

The main problem for beginning joggers is sore muscles. Even well-trained athletes sometimes double over, clutching spastic muscles after going all-out in a mile race. Effectively warming up can minimize problems for beginners.

Jogging works the buttocks, the hamstrings, and the calves in addition to the cardiovascular pulmonary system. You must stretch the leg and back muscles to prevent tightness. This is accomplished by stretching the Achilles tendon (between the calf and ankle) and the hamstring at the back of the upper leg. Always hold your stretch for a few seconds. Never bounce. Also, don't forget the front muscles—the stomach, thighs, and shins.

If you're jogging and experience a cramp or pain, use common sense—stop. Do not try to work through the pain. Massage the affected area. It should alleviate most of the cramping and soreness. If the pain persists after several days, see your physician. The main thing to remember is that if you continually experience sore muscles or cramps, you are not warming up properly.

Some people are so out of shape that they should warm up before getting out of bed. It's not as funny as it sounds. Animals, unless frightened, stretch and yawn before moving from their sleeping spot. Establish a "getting-out-of-bed" routine. Never jump out of bed. While still in bed stretch the spine, warm it up, pull your knees up to your chest, take some deep breaths, think of your happy goals; it really starts the day in an agreeable fashion. Make sure you're in touch with your whole body before rising slowly.

TIPS FOR BEGINNING JOGGERS

1. See your doctor for a comprehensive physical examination.
2. Purchase a good pair of running shoes and comfortable attire.
3. Warm up before you start.
4. Avoid running on pavement when possible. Jog on grassy surfaces. Jogging on the beach is fine but requires more stamina. Avoid running along inclines.
5. Begin by alternating jogging and walking. Jog for one minute, walk for one minute. Take it slow and easy until you build endurance. Don't push yourself.
6. Regulate your breathing. Inhale through the nose, exhale through the mouth.
7. Your jogging rhythm should be graceful, fluid.
8. To get the most out of your jogging program, spend at least thirty minutes a day, three times a week.
9. Establish reasonable goals for your program. As you attain them, set new ones.
10. Buy a good book describing the fundamentals of jogging.

JOGGING ATTIRE

The need for a good running shoe cannot be overemphasized. Shoes for jogging provide support to the heel and have flexibility. When you jog most of the stress is absorbed by the front third of your foot. That's where the shoe needs a smooth, easy bend. It is also important that the shoe be well cushioned to temper the shock to your legs and back as your feet contact the ground. Don't jog in tennis shoes. Buy jogging shoes. They're well worth the investment.

The thing to keep in mind about clothing is comfort. Forget the attractive jogging suit that binds at the crotch or the waistband. You're out there to jog, not to audition for a role in Saturday Night Fever. Also, make sure the clothes you buy are absorbent. Exercise suits that are made specifically for exercise are your best bet. They come in all price ranges and it is not imperative to spend a lot of money. In fact, a comfortable pair of shorts and an old T-shirt are perfectly adequate.

The same kinds of clothing apply equally for women. However, firm support for the breasts is absolutely essential. This can be easily accomplished by wearing a close-fitting bra with nonelastic straps or a bikini top that will provide the resistance needed. Remember, once the delicate tissue that supports the breasts is damaged, no amount of exercise can rebuild it. To avoid "jogger's nipple," irritation caused by the rubbing of nipples against rough clothing, use a strip or adhesive over each nipple. For exercising in the house or in organized classes, we recommend leotards. Make sure you buy the type with some kind of support in it. The nice thing about leotards is they look good, feel good, and make you want to exercise.

ALTERNATIVES TO JOGGING

Some of you just don't like to jog. Maybe you prefer competitive sports. Different strokes for different folks, right? That's what we've been emphasizing all along—finding what pleases you. So get out there on the tennis courts, shoot some baskets, play racquetball, join a soccer club. If you shy away from competition, go roller skating, take a swim, hike, ride a bicycle. If it's action you want, go to a disco and dance up a storm. As the saying goes, "You only go around once in life"—have fun! All of the above "pleasure" activities exercise the muscles and burn up calories. They keep you fit. Use your imagination. The possibilities for pleasure activities are virtually endless.

Remember, it's a good idea to warm up—even before stepping out onto the dance floor.

So off your duff. Give it a whirl.

Disco Dancercises

A person who makes no mistakes does not usually make anything.

⑨ Disco Dancercises

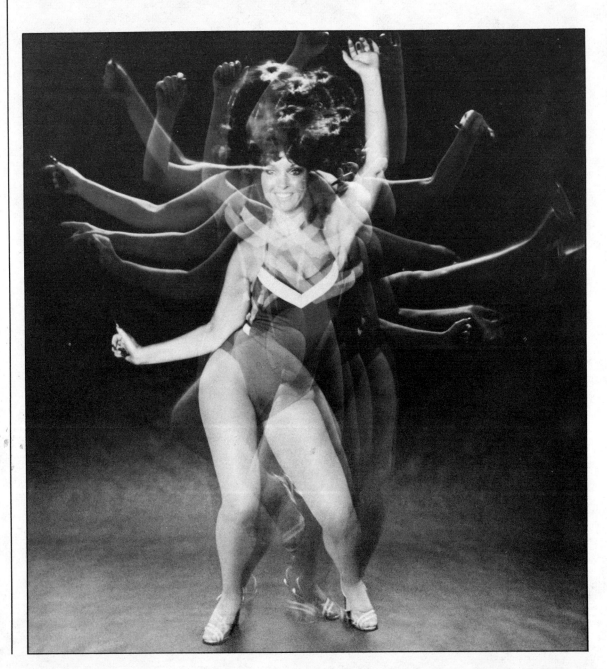

For all disco dancercises use whatever disco music you are comfortable with, preferably at an easy tempo.

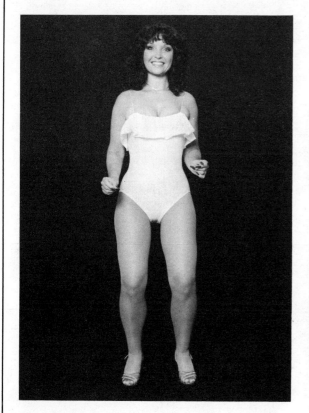
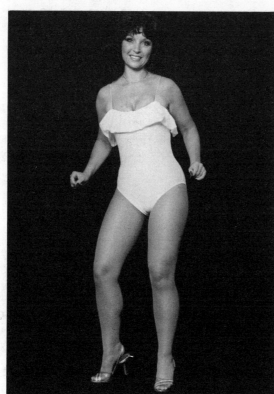
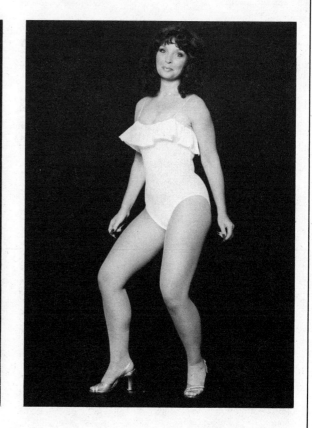

DISCO

Knee Bends (exercises top of thigh)

Standing with knees bent, bounce for 4 counts,
turn right, bounce for 4 counts. Return to the
center, bounce for 4 counts, turn left, bounce
for 4 counts. Do as many as you enjoy.

9 Disco Dancercises

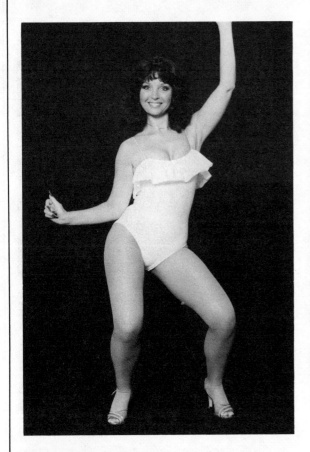 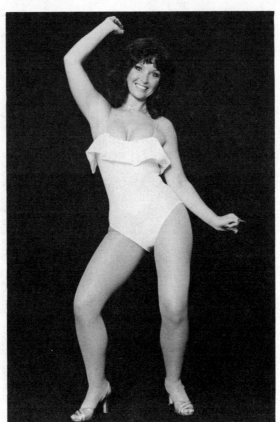

Elbow-Hip—Single and Double (exercises waist, hips, and thighs)
Standing, place right elbow on right hip. Bounce 1 count, bend knees, bounce left elbow on left hip. For variation do 2 counts on each hip.

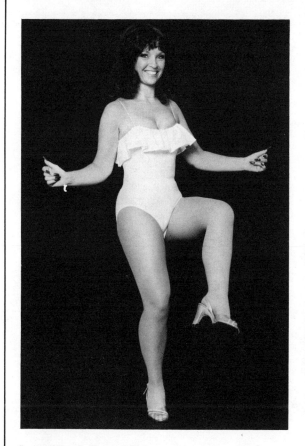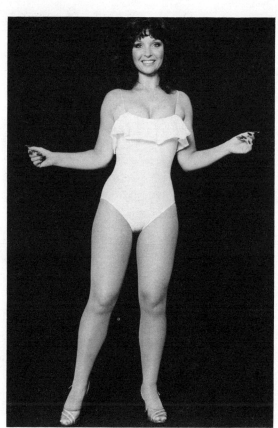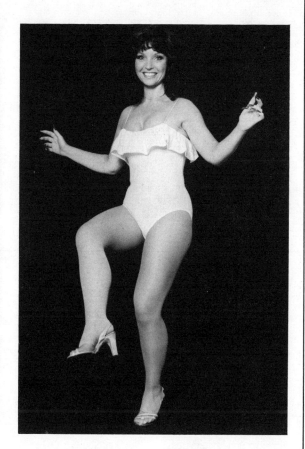

Inner Thigh Knee Lift (exercises inner thigh and top of thigh)

Stand with legs apart, bend knees. Now step right with right foot and lift left foot, heel extended, knee turned out. Use inner thigh muscle to lift leg up. Then step left and lift right leg. Keep doing this side to side for as long as you wish.

⑨ Disco Dancercises

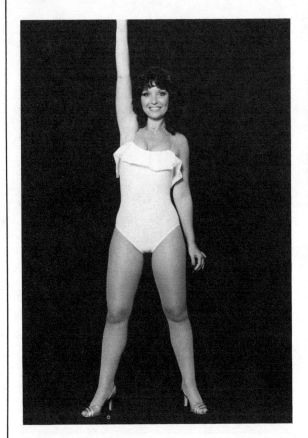
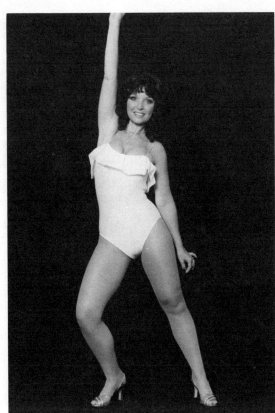
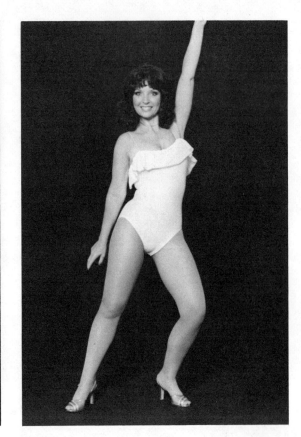

2-Count Lunges (exercises arms, waist, hips, and thighs)
Stand with legs apart, face forward, bend right knee while reaching up with right arm stretching, and bounce for 2 counts, then lunge left, bounce, and stretch for 2 counts. Do as many as you like.

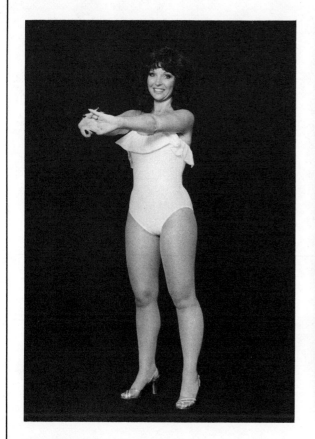
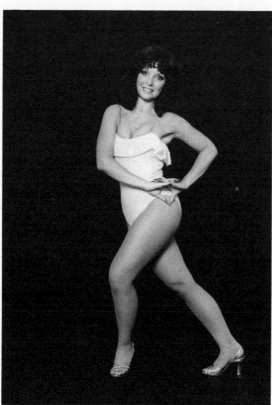
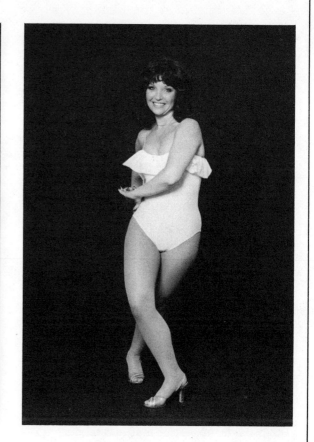

Step Back Waist Twist (exercises waist, hips, and thighs)

Stand face forward, hands clasped together, palms turned out. Take right foot and cross behind left foot and at the same time bring hands across body to left side of waist. Now step back with left foot and bring hands to right side of waist. Repeat. Do as many as you wish.

⑨ Disco Dancercises

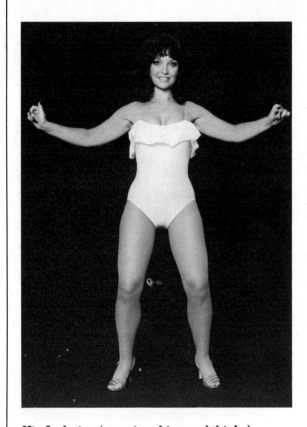 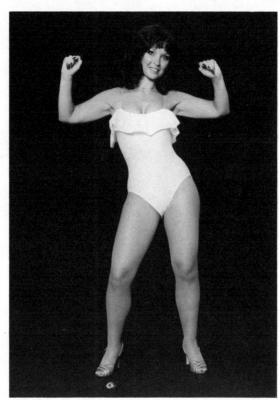 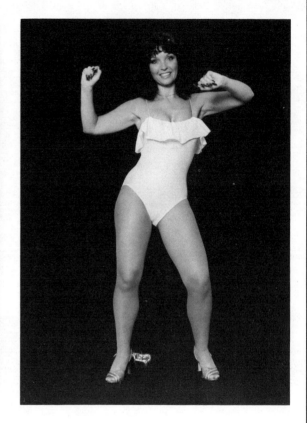

Hip Isolation (exercises hips and thighs)
Stand with feet apart, bend knees, now move
only the hips from right to left. Tighten the
buttock on the side you lean toward. This
makes the hip snap from side to side. For
variety do 2 counts on each side.

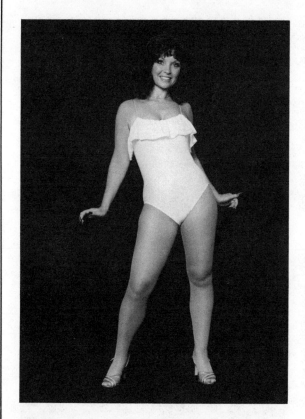
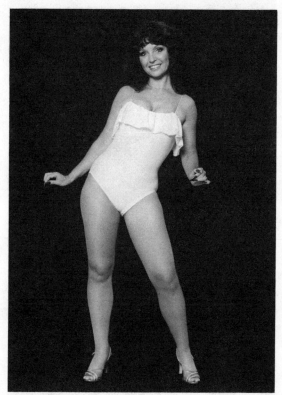

Hip Swing (exercises hips, buttocks, and thighs)
Stand with feet apart and swing hips from side to side trying to bump an invisible wall. Move each side alternately. For variety do 2 counts on each side movement.

9 Disco Dancercises

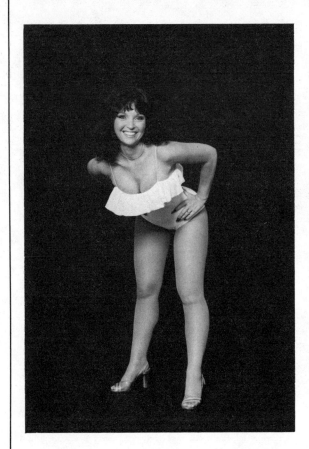

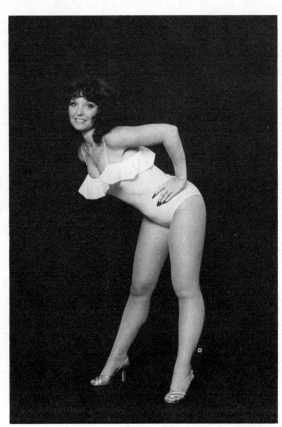

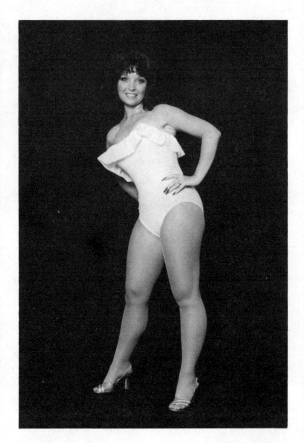

One-Half Hip Circle (exercises hips, thighs, and buttocks)

Stand with feet apart, bend torso forward, swing hips in a half-circle to the right, and stop. Now swing hips in a half-circle to the left side. Do as many as you like.

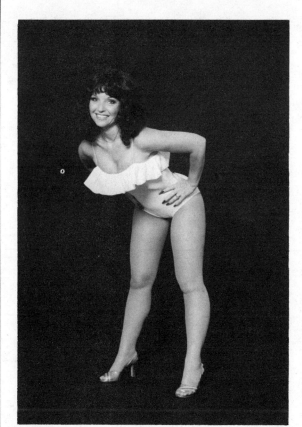
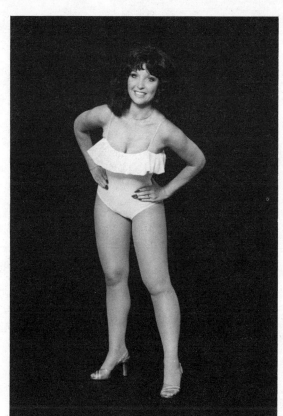
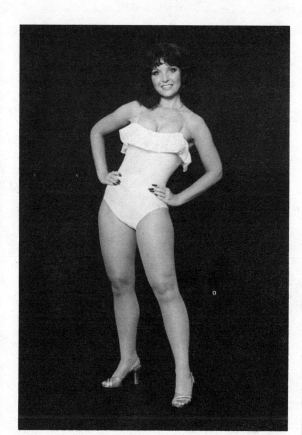

⑨ Disco Dancercises

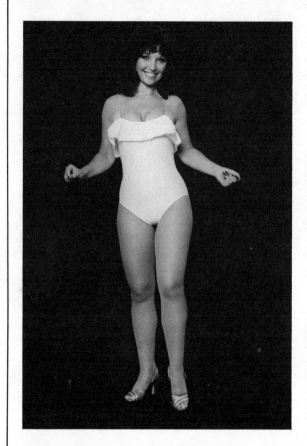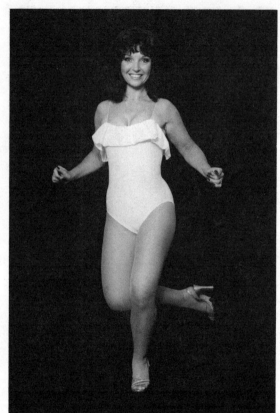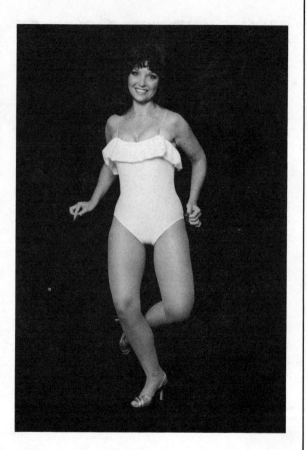

Step Kick Back (exercises back of thigh)
Stand, step forward with the right foot, and
kick the left foot back. Now step left and kick
right foot back. Do as many times as you wish.

Daily Dozens

"Happiness is not being pained in body or troubled in mind."
Thomas Jefferson

FOR WOMEN

Daily Dozens should become the exercising
bible for women. As the name implies, they
should be done on a daily basis. You've gotten
into the habit of brushing your teeth and comb-
ing your hair. Why not get into the Daily
Dozens habit? Incorporate them into your life-
style. It will be the most beneficial program
you can adopt.

Follow the calendar in the front of the
book. Be good to yourself and take the time to
do something for you. The results will carry
over to other aspects of your life. You'll become
a more positive, uplifting, relaxed person.

Be fun to be around. It can't hurt to try.

FOR MEN

The majority of today's men still function in
the traditional role of the family breadwinner.
By taking care of yourself, you are expressing
your love for your family. You are showing
them that you want to be around to enjoy life
with them—be a part of their future. Your daily
dozens may change the atmosphere in your
home from negative to positive.

Remember, a positive mental attitude goes
hand in hand with a healthy, fit body.

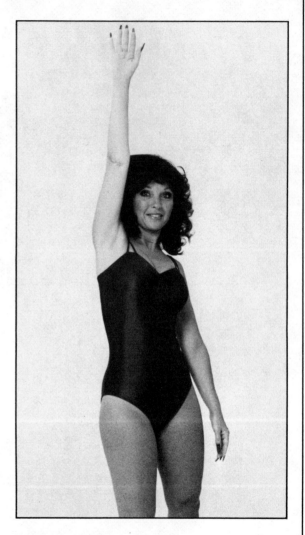

DAILY DOZENS—WOMEN

Stretch and Reach (warm-up)
Stand with feet apart, raise one arm toward
ceiling and exhale. Reach for ceiling with the
other arm as you drop first arm, and inhale at
the same time. Repeat 10 to 20 times. Really
stretch and reach.

Push-Ups (exercises bust and arms)
Start on hands and knees, palms flat, elbows
straight. Slowly lower body to the floor, bend
elbows. Do not touch the floor. Then push up
slowly by straightening elbows. Inhale on the
way down, exhale as you push up. Start with
10 reps, work up to 20 reps a day before
advancing to men's push-ups.

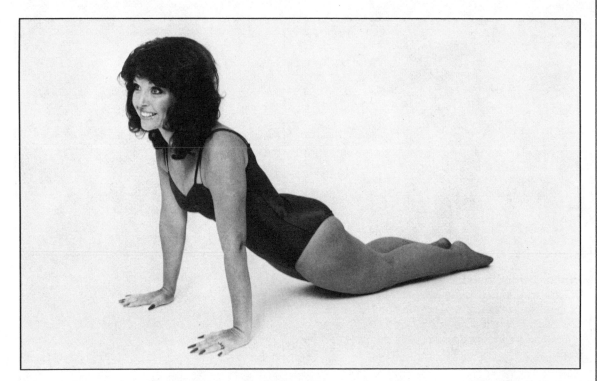

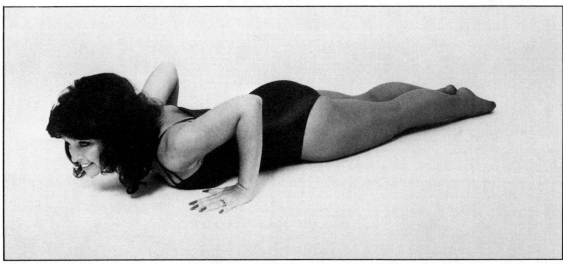

78

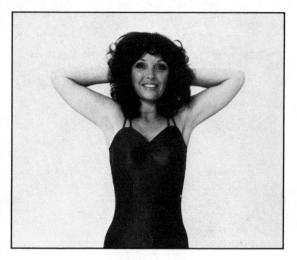

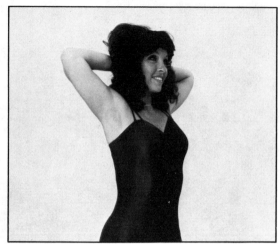

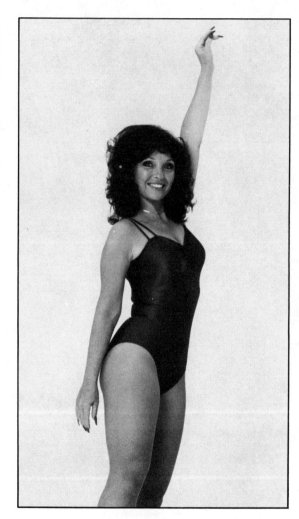

Hands Behind Head Waist Twist
Stand with legs apart, unlock knees, squeeze buttocks together. Place hands behind head. Twist from side to side. Inhale at center, exhale on twist. Beginners do 10 reps, work up to 50 reps.

Alternate Side Bend Press
Stand with legs apart, squeeze buttocks together, unlock knees, pull stomach in. Place right elbow on right hip, left arm straight over head. Bend to right. Then change sides and bend to left with left elbow on left hip and right arm straight up. Exhale on each stretch. Start with 10, work up to 30.

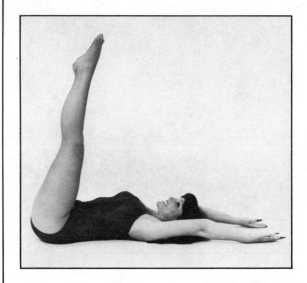

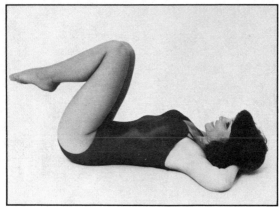

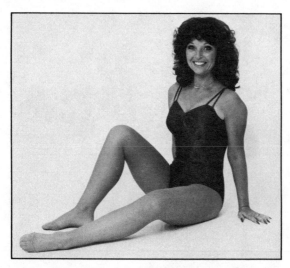

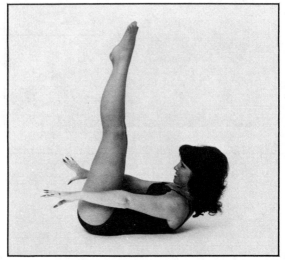

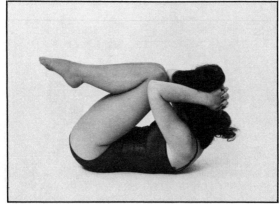

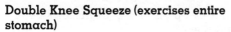

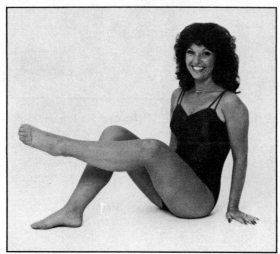

Wall Sit-Up (exercises stomach muscles)

Lie on your back with legs straight up in the air, arms overhead, and inhale. Now bring hands past legs while exhaling. Return to floor and repeat. Beginners do 10 reps, work up to 50 reps a day.

Double Knee Squeeze (exercises entire stomach)

Lie on floor, hands behind head, bend knees. Bring head and shoulders up off floor and squeeze knees with elbows. Inhale on starting position, exhale on squeeze. Do 10 reps one side and repeat on other side. Work up to 50 reps on each side.

Inner Thigh Slice

Sit on the floor, pull stomach in, bend one knee. The other leg is slightly bent on the floor with knee turned out. Now inhale and lift the leg in a slicing motion up to bent knee while exhaling. Beginners do 10 reps on each side, work up to 20 reps.

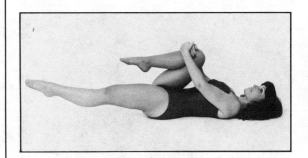

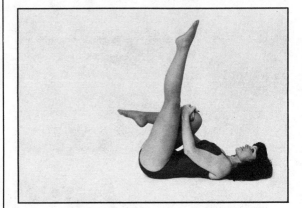

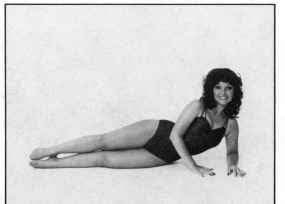

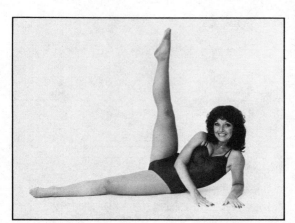

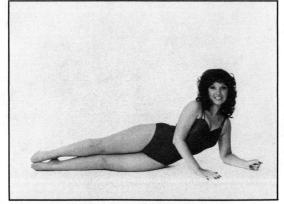

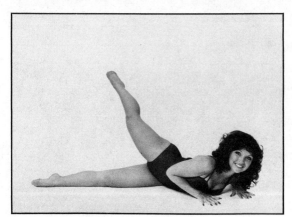

Hold One Knee Leg Lift (exercises top of thigh)
Lie on back, hold one knee, other leg is
straight. Inhale. Lift leg and exhale at same
time. Repeat on other side. Beginners do 10
reps on each side, work up to 50 reps each
side.

**Side Leg Kick-Up and Back (exercises side of
thigh and buttocks)**
Lie on side, bring straight leg to shoulder, and
exhale. Roll a little forward, inhale, kick back,
and exhale. Repeat on other side. Beginners
do 10 on each side, work up to 20 reps per side.

Side Knee-Up Straight Leg-Up (exercises hips and thighs)

Lie on left side, legs together and straight. Recline on left elbow, right hand in front of body for support. Inhale and bring knee up to shoulder, exhale, then straight back down and inhale, then back up to shoulder with straight leg and exhale. Repeat on other side. Do 10 reps on each side, work up to 20 reps.

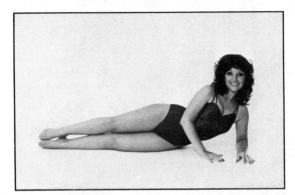

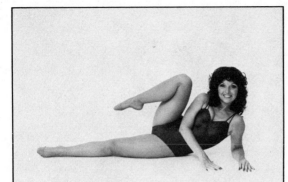

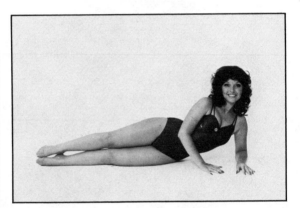

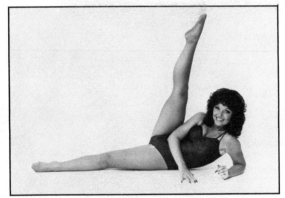

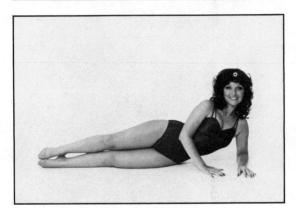

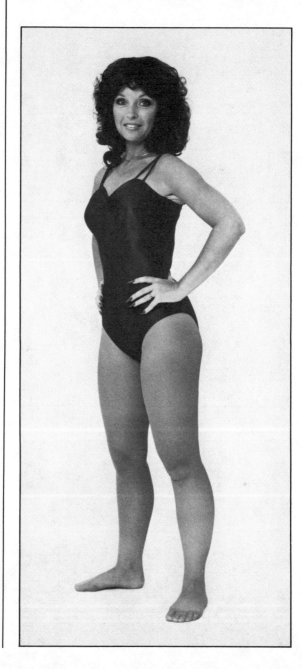

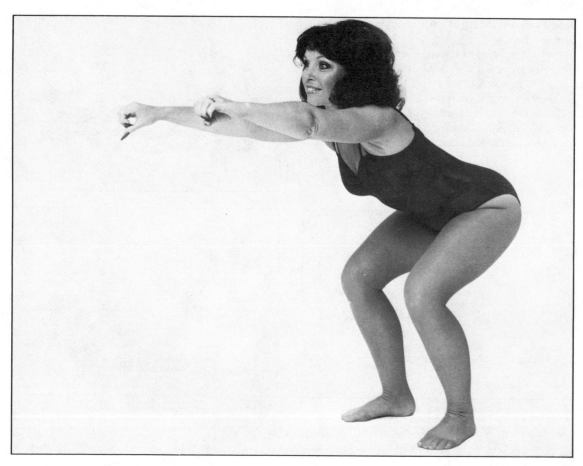

Pivot Point Knee Bend (exercises hips and entire thigh)

Stand with legs apart, unlock knees, reach for one wall with your hands and arms and another wall with your bottom. (Do not do a knee bend.) Return to starting position. Inhale at starting position, exhale as you reach forward. This exercise is excellent for working hips and thighs without hurting the lower back or placing stress on the knees. Beginners do 10 reps, work up to 50 reps.

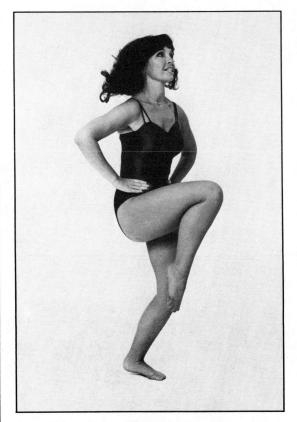
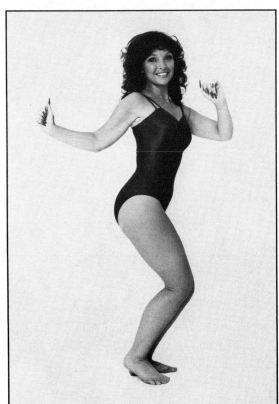
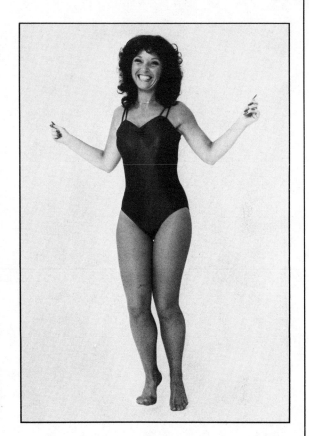

Jog in Place, Jump Waist Twist, or Rope Jump (exercises cardiovascular and pulmonary system—heart, blood vessels, and lungs)

For jump waist twist, stand with feet together, knees bent, jump and point knees to the left. Twist torso and arms to the right. Continue alternating 10 times. Work up to 50 times.

For rope jump, jump as if you are using a jump rope. If you have a jump rope, use it. Jump 10 times, and work up to 50.

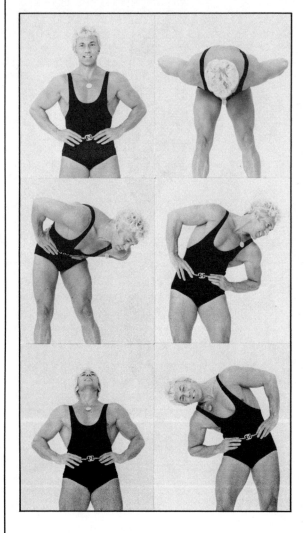

DAILY DOZENS—MEN

Torso Circle (warm-up for torso)

Stand with legs apart, unlock knees, pull stomach in, inhale, bend forward at waist, and exhale. Roll to the right side, then to the back, then to the left side, and return to center. Exhale. Do 10 one way and 10 the other way. Exhale when you bend forward. Inhale on the upswing.

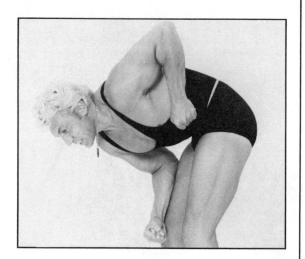

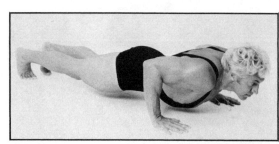

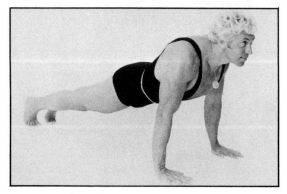

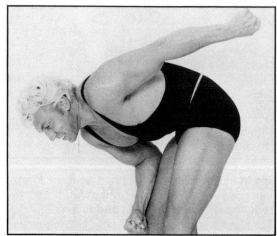

Push-Up

Hands on floor, palms flat, back is flat, legs straight, toes touching floor. Inhale down, exhale as you push up. Start with 10 reps, work up to 50 a day.

Triceps Extension (exercises back of arm)

Stand with feet apart, bend over until torso and upper arm are parallel to floor. Straighten arm until forearm is also parallel. Tense triceps, lower arm, and repeat. Do 10 reps and increase as is comfortable.

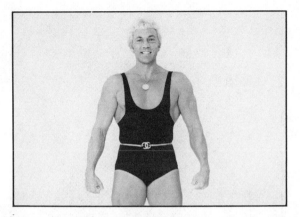

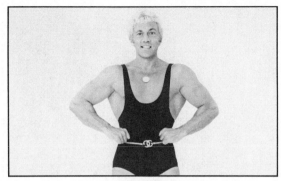

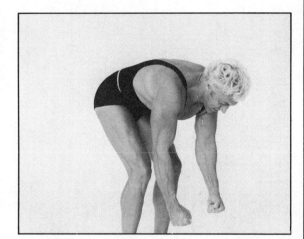

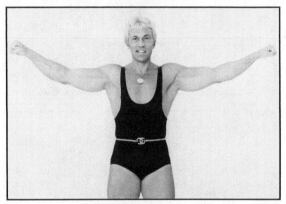

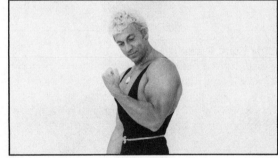

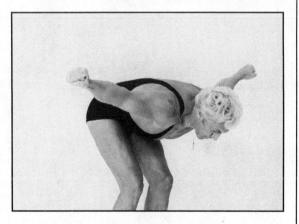

Delt Raise (exercises shoulder—deltoid muscle)
Stand with feet apart, raise straight arms until slightly above parallel to floor. Tense shoulder muscles, lower, and repeat. Beginners do 10 reps, increase as is comfortable.

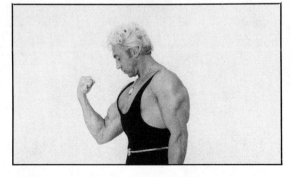

Curls (exercises front of arm—biceps muscle)
Stand with legs apart, palms up. Make fists, bend arms until fists touch shoulders. Tense biceps, lower, and repeat. Beginners do 10 reps, increase as is comfortable.

Bent Over Side Raise (exercises back muscles)
Stand with legs apart, bend over from waist. Raise arms until slightly above parallel to floor, pause for a second, contract back muscles, lower arms back to starting position. Beginners do 10 reps, increase as is comfortable.

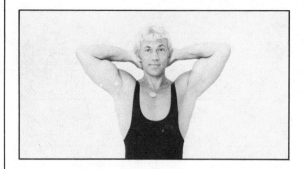

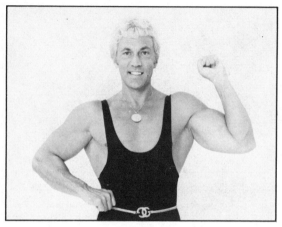

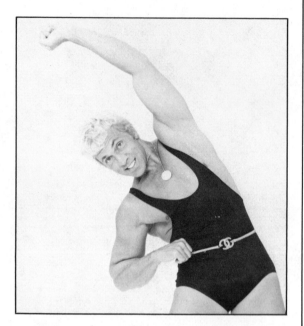

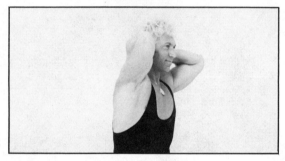

Side Bend Press
Standing with legs apart, place right elbow on right hip, left arm straight over head. Bend to side. Then change sides and bend to side with left elbow on left hip and right arm straight up. Beginners do 10, work up to 30.

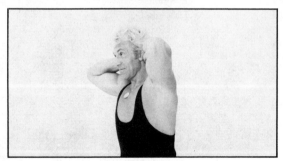

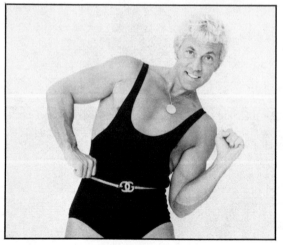

Hand Behind Head Waist Twist
Stand with legs apart, place hands behind head. Twist from side to side. Inhale at center, exhale on twist. Beginners do 20 reps, work up to 50 reps.

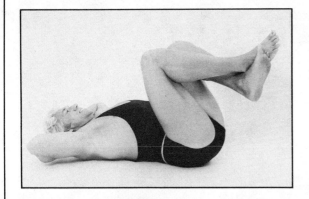

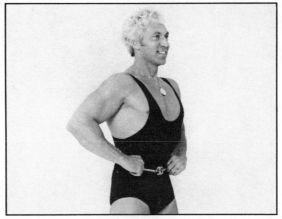

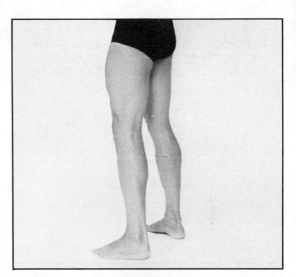

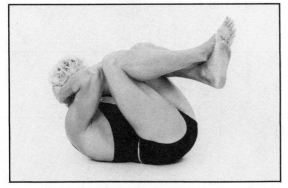

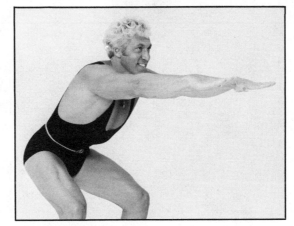

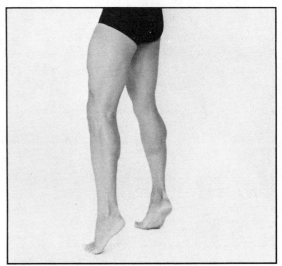

Quarter Sit-Up (works entire stomach)
Lie on floor, bend knees, hands behind head, and inhale. Now exhale and touch elbows to knees. Do this exercise at a good pace and with a smooth rhythm. Always exhale on stomach squeeze. Beginners do 10, work up to 50.

Pivot Point Knee Bend (exercises hips and entire thigh)
Stand with legs apart, squeeze buttocks, unlock knees. Reach for one wall with your hands and arms and another wall with your bottom. (Do not do a knee bend.) Then return to starting position. Inhale at starting position, exhale as you reach forward. This exercise is excellent for working hips and thighs without hurting the lower back or placing stress on the knees. Beginners do 10 reps, work up to 50.

Calf Raise
Stand with feet apart. (Beginners hold on to a chair for balance.) Inhale, rise up on toes, exhale. Return to starting position. Beginners do 10 reps, work up to as many as you can do.

88

High Knee Jog

Fast jog—try to bring knees to waist level for
10 counts. Breathe normally and jog in place
moving quickly. Set your own limit but don't
overdo.

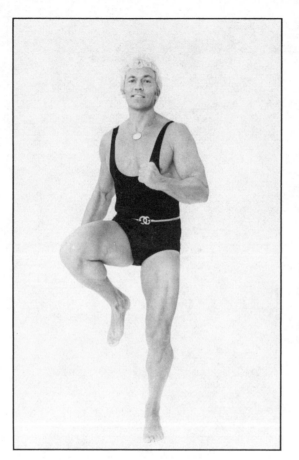
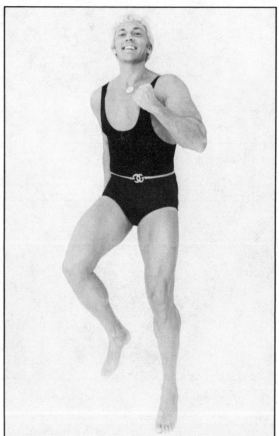

11

Resistance Exercises

"We undo ourselves by impatience.
Misfortunes have their life and their limits."
Michel de Montaigne

90 Resistance can be defined as a counterforce to your exercise activity. Most people relate this to some form of lifting weights—"pumping iron." However, as a beginner, you can select almost any object that can be easily found in the house. Cans of soup, pots with handles, plastic detergent bottles with handles provide resistance. Pulling at either end of a towel tightens the muscles and offers resistance. To progress on your exercise program you must utilize resistance.

When you start your routine of calisthenics, your body weight provides the resistance. Your resistance increases with the number of repetitions and the speed with which you do the exercise. However, this resistance will diminish as you firm up your body weight and grow stronger. Thus, at some point you should use a weighted object as your resistance. The more resistance, the faster the results. However, make sure you build up resistance slowly. Don't start by picking up a fifty-pound barbell —that's too much resistance for a beginner. Progress at a comfortable rate so that you don't hurt yourself.

RESISTANCE

For a little extra resistance, use cans, weights, or fill plastic bottles that have handles with sand or water or even kitty litter.

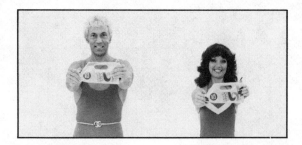

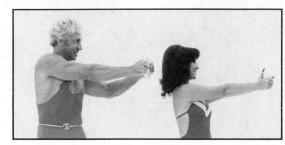

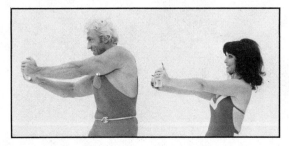

Two-Hand Waist Twist (exercises waist)
Stand with legs apart, place one hand on each end of plastic bottle, inhale, and exhale as you twist to the right. Return to the center position. Inhale, twist left, and exhale. Beginners do 10 reps, work up to 50 reps.

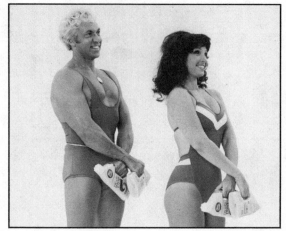

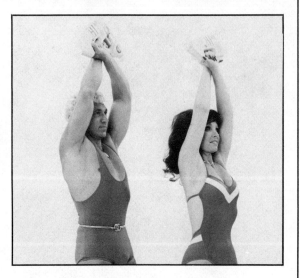

Wrist Cross Overhead (exercises bustline, chest, and shoulders)
Stand with legs apart. Hold a plastic bottle in each hand, cross wrists at the lap, inhale. Now bring arms overhead, cross wrist, and exhale. Repeat movement. Beginners do 10, work up to 20 reps.

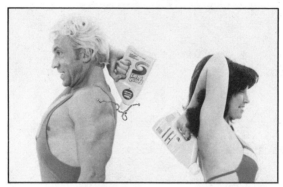

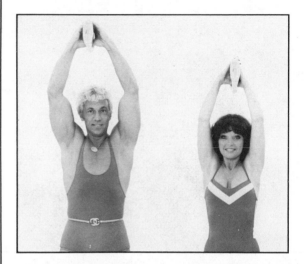

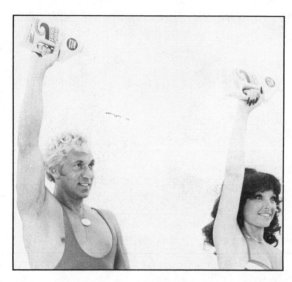

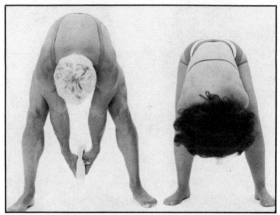

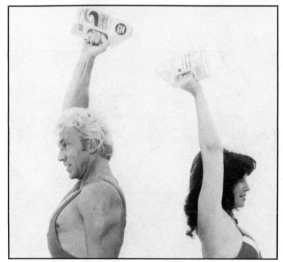

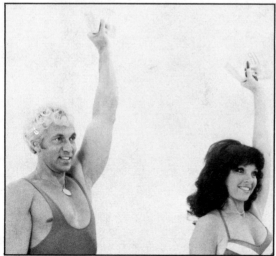

Wood Chop (exercises hips, thighs, buttocks, chest, arms, waist, stomach)

Stand with legs apart, unlock knees, pull stomach in. Place hands on plastic bottle and swing up over your head while inhaling. Swing bottle down through legs while exhaling and bending knees. Beginners do 10 reps, work up to 50 reps.

Overhead Triceps Extension (exercises back of arm)

Standing, place plastic bottle in left hand, arm bent and against side of head, and inhale. Extend arm up and exhale. Beginners do 10 reps each side, work up to 50 reps for each side.

Arm Changes (exercises shoulders)

Stand with legs apart. Put a plastic bottle in each hand. Inhale and bring one arm up and exhale. Repeat with other arm. Do 10 reps, work up to 50 reps.

11 Resistance Exercises

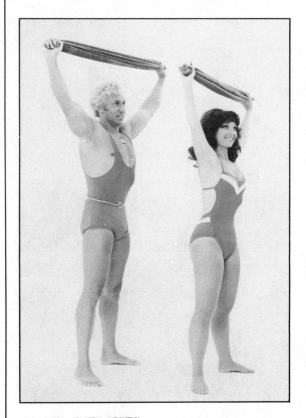 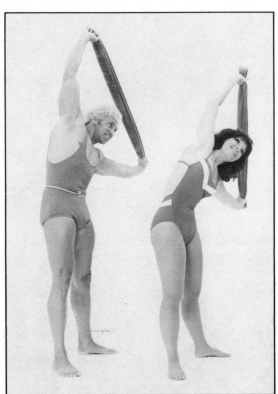 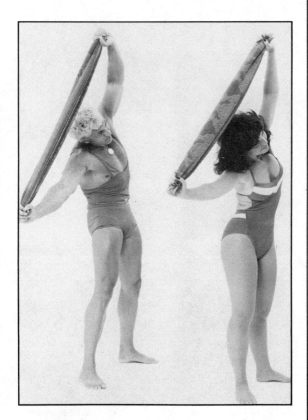

TOWEL EXERCISES

Side-Center-Side Bends (for waistline)

Stand with legs apart, tighten buttocks, pull
stomach in, and unlock knees. Grasp a rolled-
up towel with both hands, keeping hands as
far apart as possible. Raise towel above your
head, inhale and bend torso to the left, arms
straight. Return to center position and exhale.
Inhale and bend to the right, straighten up and
exhale. Do 10 reps on each side, continuing
slowly until you can do 20 reps.

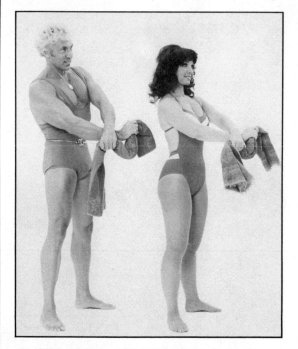

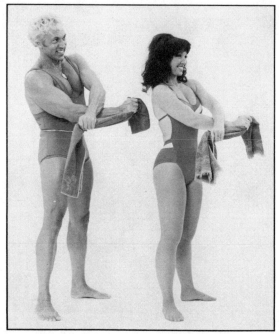

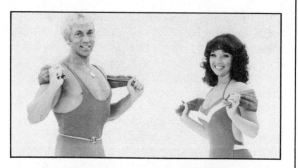

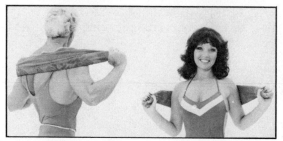

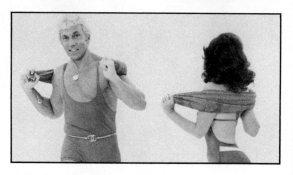

Pectoral Pull (for bustline)

Stand with legs apart. Grasp one end of the towel with the right hand, cross the left hand over the right hand, grasp the other end of the towel, and inhale. With a sharp snapping motion, push hands farther across chest and exhale. Do 10 reps, working up to 20 reps.

Waist Twist (for waistline)

Stand with legs apart, tighten buttocks, pull stomach in, unlock knees. Place rolled-up towel around top of back, holding towel tightly with both hands, and inhale. Twist to the left without moving feet and exhale. Return to center position, then twist to the right. From left twist to right twist is a continuous motion. Do 10 reps to the left and 10 to the right, slowly work up to 50 reps.

94

Running Lunge (for cardiovascular system, hips, and thighs)

Stand with legs apart, rolled-up towel held in both hands as far apart as possible, arms straight and overhead. Inhale. As you begin to lunge forward, keep right leg on floor and straight. As the left leg goes forward, bend the left knee (one giant step movement). Exhale on lunge. Move back to standing position and reverse leg movement (right leg forward, left leg back and straight). Beginners do 10 reps, work up to 50. Arms may get tired at first, so do only as many of the running lunge as comfortable.

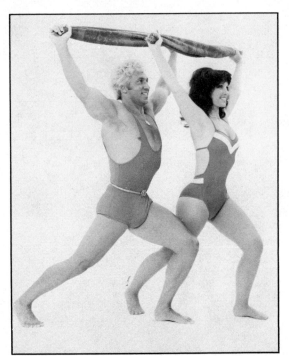
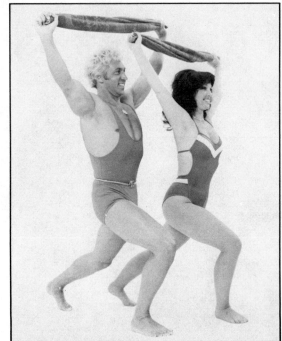

12

Senior Citizens

12 Senior Citizens

"I'll do it tomorrow, but tomorrow never comes . . ." applies to the majority of our senior citizens who have become physically inactive. More than any other group, senior citizens need to exercise. If you are older and have allowed yourself to become sedentary, daily activities such as reaching for a can on a shelf, climbing stairs, or even rising from a chair become arduous tasks. It takes so little effort to begin a fitness program. Stamp your feet, lift your arms, twist your body, move your head in a circle, point your toes. You're on your way. If you keep it up, your progress will surprise you.

The "Body Buddies" concept works especially well for senior citizens who have allowed themselves to become lost in the endless hours of television game shows and soap operas. You and your buddy can take the time to walk, exercise, even jog for a while. You can select a program that will give you back your mobility and your independence. Always be sure you check with your doctor before starting.

SENIOR CITIZENS

The following exercises are designed to keep the blood circulating and to activate unused muscles. Practice them slowly at first.

Handshake and Massage (brings circulation to hands)

Seated in a chair, shake your hands 10 times. Then massage palm of hand with thumb and forefinger starting at the top of the palm and working toward the fingertip of each finger. Do as many as you like.

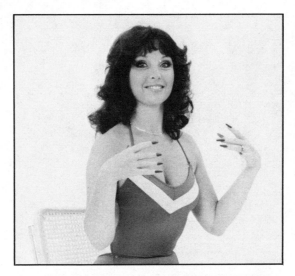
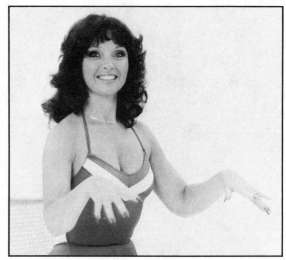
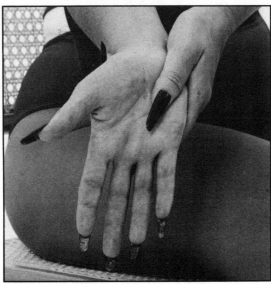
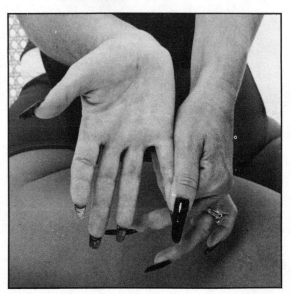

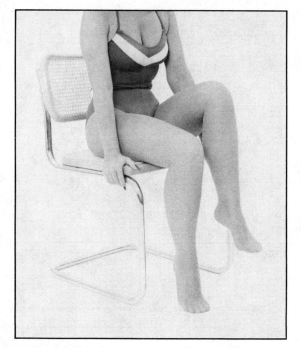
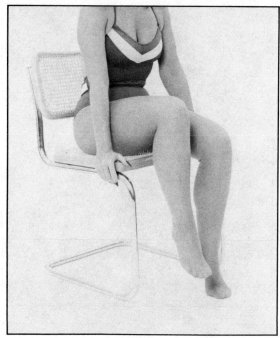
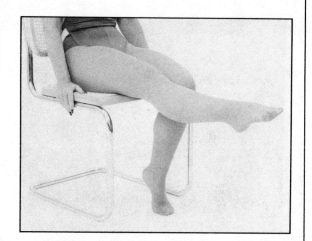
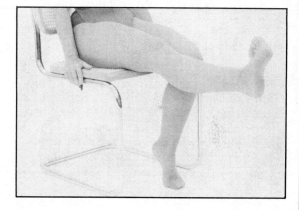

Chair Stomp (brings circulation to the lower leg)
Seated in a chair, move legs alternately up and down slowly. Do as many times a day as comfortable.

Calf Push (for calf, ankle, and front of lower leg)
Seated in a chair, point toe, then extend heel. Beginners do 10 times or as many as you wish.

Single Leg Pull
Lie on the floor, legs straight. Inhale and raise one knee toward your chest, hold knee for a second. Lower leg and exhale. Raise the opposite leg, inhale up, exhale down. Do 10 reps or only as many as comfortable. (Not shown.)

12 *Senior Citizens*

98

"I DON'T HAVE THE TIME"

How many times have you heard that excuse? How many times have you said it yourself? What the statement really means is, "I won't take the time to help myself." In this world we occupy temporarily, time is our most important commodity. In fact, all we really have is time. When we won't take the time to exercise and become healty, fit human beings, it diminishes our time on this planet.

So loosen your grip on this negative attitude. Say to yourself, "I must take the time," "I must exercise," "I must do something for me." You've got nothing to lose, everything to gain. Time cannot be recalled or recycled— but **you** can be.

Ready to make that commitment? Good!

CHAIR

Dips (works back of arm)
Beginners place hands on front of chair, bend knees under you as if you're sitting on your heels. Inhale and press up until arms are straight and exhale. Drop back down and inhale. Do 10 reps, work up to 50 reps.

Knee-Ups (works stomach)
Sit on front part of chair seat with legs straight out and hands holding edge of chair. Inhale, then bring knees to chest and exhale. Return legs to floor. Repeat 10 times, work up to 20 reps.

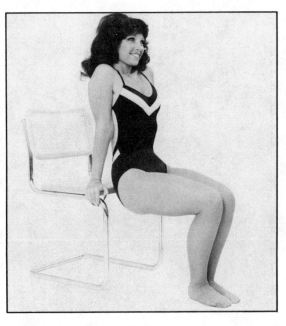

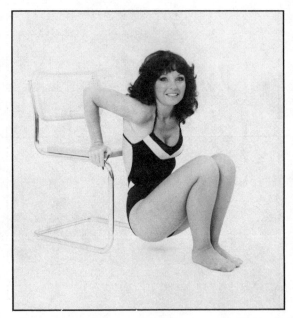

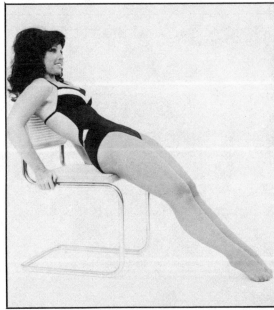

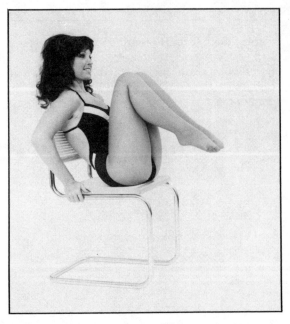

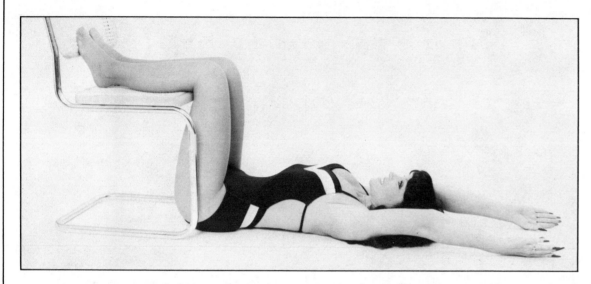

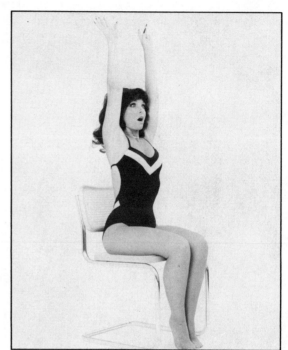

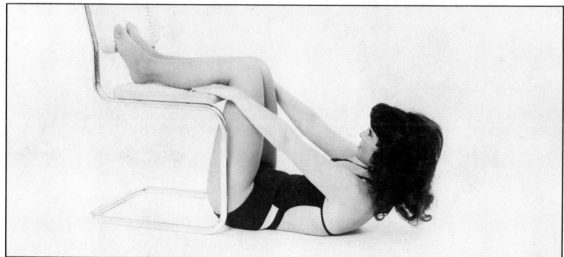

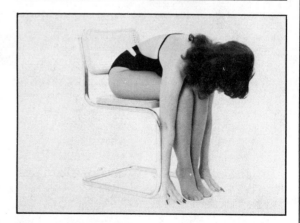

Bent Knee Chair Sit-Up (works stomach)
Lie on the floor, place legs on seat of chair
with arms overhead. Inhale and curl body to
chair while exhaling. Bring hands up and over
to touch chair seat. Return to starting position.
Do 10 times, work up to 50 reps.

Inhale—Exhale
Sit on a chair and raise both arms overhead
while inhaling deeply. Bring arms down, touch
the floor and exhale. Do 10 reps only.

12 Senior Citizens

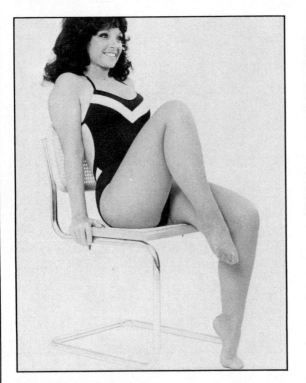

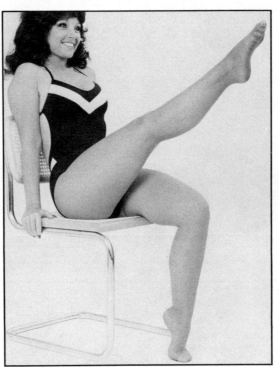

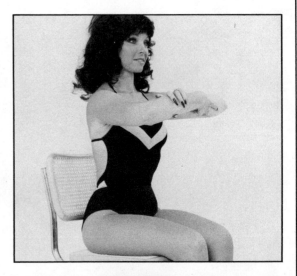

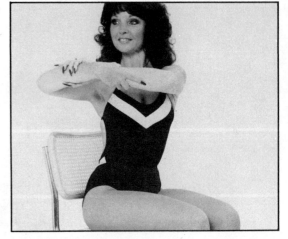

Side Bend, Arms Overhead (exercises the waist)

Sit on a chair, interlock fingers while keeping arms straight out in front of you. In one motion, face palms of hands away from you and raise arms overhead. Inhale deeply, bend torso to the left and exhale. Straighten up, inhale, then bend to the right and exhale. Beginners do 10 reps, work up to 20 reps. (Not shown.)

One Knee In, Out, and Down (exercises top of thigh)

Sit in chair and hold on to the sides of the chair. Inhale and bring right knee up to chest, keeping left leg on the floor. Exhale and reverse process, left knee up, right leg down. Beginners do 10 reps each side, work up to 20 reps for each side.

Forearm Waist Twist (exercises the waist)

While seated in a chair, raise arms and clasp each forearm with hands, inhale and twist upper torso to the left. Your feet should be firmly planted on the floor. Return to center position, inhale, twist to the right and exhale. Do 10 reps on each side, slowly progressing to 20 reps.

13

Nutritional Soundings

13 Nutritional Soundings

Nutrition determines the way you look, act, and feel. Poor nutrition, coupled with inactivity, can make you listless, grouchy, and not very good company. Conversely, proper nutrition can make your cheeks rosy, create a glow around you, and make your personality attractive to others. The majority of people who enter exercise programs are overweight—the victims of too many gourmet meals, too much pie, cakes, candy, and ice cream. So let's start eating right, okay?

REDUCING

The choice of foods is the most important factor in reducing. A balanced diet with plenty of variety is the key. And remember, calories do count. Too little food reduces nutritional intake below acceptable levels. Too much food won't allow you to lose weight rapidly enough to suit your desires.

Once you've committed yourself to a program of weight loss, stick with it. Like exercising, you have to set up the diet program that's right for you. Consult with a good nutritionist or your personal physician before starting your program.

A simple rule for good nutrition is to have protein as the basis of each meal, along with limited amounts of food containing carbohydrates.

Use of food and vitamin supplements insures adequate nutrition. Absolutely **no** refined foods should be eaten. These are foods that contain sugar or white flour. Also, avoid preservatives, colorings, and other unnatural additives. Here is a sample of a well-balanced menu for weight reduction.

Breakfast	Calories	Protein	Carbo-hydrates	Fat
2 poached, soft boiled, hard boiled, or fried (no oil) eggs	160	12	0.8	12
½ glass lowfat milk	70	5	7	2.5
½ slice whole grain wheat toast	32.5	1.5	5.5	.5
w/butter	60	0	0	6.5
½ cantaloupe	35	1	8	0
Total	357.5	19.5	21.3	21.5
Lunch				
Salad (2 cups)	65	4	8	0
Apple cider vinegar (2 Tbsp.) and safflower oil dressing (1 Tbsp.)	120	0	0	13
3 oz. tuna	170	25	0	17
Total	355	29	8	30
Dinner				
8 oz. broiled chicken	225	23	0	14
4 oz. green beans	30	2	6	0
½ slice whole grain wheat toast	32.5	1.5	5.5	0.5
	287.5	26.5	11.5	14.5
Total for day	1,000	75	40.8	66
Goals for day	1,000 to 1,200	65 to 100	40 to 60	50 to 70

If you follow this type of menu, you'll soon see the pounds disappear. And guess what? You're not even starving yourself.

Jeanne prefers the following foods in her favorite weight reduction program.

Breakfast: Complete Protein Concentrate Shake. 8 oz. nonfat milk in blender. Start blender, add 2 Tbsp. complete protein powder, blend approximately ½ minute. Options: ice cubes (3 or 4) for thickness and chill, or add nutmeg or cinnamon on top for flavor, or blend ¼ banana for flavor.
A natural vitamin and mineral supplement.

Lunch: Eat and enjoy as much as you like of the following: Chef salad with tuna, turkey, or chicken. Use vinegar/oil or lemon/oil dressing.

Dinner: 4-6 oz. protein such as chicken, fish, tuna, or turkey. Fresh vegetables, ½ slice whole grain wheat bread, 1 glass nonfat milk.

For more rapid reducing, omit the evening meal and have a protein drink instead (the same as you would for breakfast). Also, take a natural vitamin and mineral supplement. Use your own judgment and find the reducing program that's right for you. It's not a sin to be thin.

MAINTENANCE DIET

Once you reach the proper body weight, you can use many of the reducing principles to maintain your new look. But it is your positive attitude that remains your greatest ally in the battle of the bulge.

Instead of viewing your new eating habits as restrictive, realize that you will deny yourself only what we call "anti-foods"—foods that either are harmful to you or don't provide nutrition. In place of these anti-foods you will eat "foods for life," which supply the body with essential nutrients, providing you with more energy by burning excess and undesirable fat in the body.

An easy way to burn fat and keep trim is to replace one meal a day with a delicious protein drink.

The basic protein drink is eight ounces of nonfat milk, or your favorite unsweetened natural fruit juice, mixed or blended with one ounce (approximately two heaping tablespoons) of high-quality milk and egg protein powder. The powder should not merely contain a high percentage of protein but should supply complete vitamins and minerals—nature's catalysts—which help the body digest and assimilate protein. It should have no sugar, dextrose, corn syrup, or other sweeteners, except honey or fructose.

For variety and a more appetizing protein shake, add any of the following to the base mix: fruit, yogurt (without sugar), bran, lecithin, brewers yeast (easy does it at first), wheat germ, sunflower seeds, sesame seeds, raw nuts or nut butters, cinnamon, or nutmeg. Make a tasty shake, but don't overdo the high-carbohydrate items such as pineapple juice (or other juices and fruits rated high in carbohydrates—you can check a carbohydrate

guide for exact amounts).

This complete shake should replace breakfast one day, lunch the next, dinner another. Using the shake in this manner will not only help control your calorie and carbohydrate intake but will change your attitude toward "three squares a day" and "meat and potatoes" meals.

The other two meals (or all three if you prefer) should include a balanced variety of fresh, natural foods from the four basic food groups. Sugar, white flour, and other processed anti-foods containing them should be avoided. Read labels. Take responsibility. Most canned and packaged foods have processed ingredients. There's virtually no need to eat something that comes in a box or a can when so much wholesome, fresh (refrigerated) food is available.

We also wholeheartedly suggest you top off each meal with a good vitamin-mineral supplement. These supplements contain natural ingredients such as desiccated liver, yeast, bone meal, kelp, alfalfa, and cod liver oil. You should spread the effectiveness of the supplement over the entire day rather than taking one tablet only once a day.

Between-meal snacks should be avoided unless they are small portions of raw vegetables or hard cheese. These snacks can help you get through "low energy" days, but don't overeat. When you must snack, eat smaller portions during your regular meals.

Follow the "foods for life" carefully. Whenever you eat, realize that food should help you maintain proper body weight, along with adding to your health and to your ability to enjoy life.

Make complete shake meals a habit and break that ritual of stuffing yourself two or three times a day. Let your eating habits remind you of the relationship between eating and your attitude toward life and happiness. They make a difference. Keep your attitudes dynamic and positive.

Eat right. Eat light. Experience the feeling of well-being that "foods for life" can put into your life.

GAINING WEIGHT

The key to all weight-gaining programs lies in exercise. A high protein, high calorie, or high-carbohydrate meal will be stored as fat unless a good exercise program is followed. It's more desirable to have muscle weight than fat weight! Gain weight, but watch your waistline.

Here are a few general rules you should follow.

1. Whether for weight gain or weight loss, you should eliminate all sugar and all products containing sugar.
2. Eat at least three well-balanced meals every day made up of the following foods:
   a. Have at least six ounces and up to one pound of any protein source at each of the three meals. Protein sources include fish, seafood, poultry, eggs, milk, cheese, and meat.
   b. Have at least two fresh fruits daily.
   c. Have at least one large raw salad daily.
   d. Have at least one cooked vegetable daily.
   e. Have no less than two, but no more than four, servings of any whole grain products.
3. Have as much milk, fruit, and vegetable juices as you wish. Omit coffee. Drink herb teas.

4. If more weight is to be gained, add food supplements and vitamins and minerals as follows:
   a. Have a complete protein concentrate drink with each meal.
   b. Have a complete protein concentrate drink between each meal, or whenever desired.
   c. Digestion-aiding tablets with each drink are recommended.
   d. Take natural vitamin and mineral supplements at each meal.

Here is a recipe for a complete protein concentrate drink:

Place in blender:
8 oz. whole milk (preferably medically certified raw)
4 rounded tbsp. milk and egg protein powder
Ice as desired
The following may be added to your drink for taste and extra calories:
1 whole fresh fruit (banana, apple, strawberries, etc.)
1 tbsp. honey
Honey ice cream (no sugar)
Yogurt (no sugar), natural peanut butter
Cinnamon, nutmeg, and other spices
Carob powder

All protein drinks should be consumed slowly and never gulped. It is important that all foods are digested properly so that the maximum amount of nutrients is obtained. Happy eating!

CONCLUSION

It's now time for you to sit down (we'd prefer that you stand) and plan your new program of exercise and nutrition. Remember, plan one that is suited to your individual needs and desires. Plan it together with your husband, wife, friend, or lover. The Body Buddies concept makes physical fitness fun. Set goals for yourself. Let your body buddy know your goals. Make your commitment to health. Remember, don't make your goals too ambitious. Once you've decided on your program, stick with it.

If you follow the instructions in this book, you'll be amazed at how good you'll feel, how much vitality and zest will have returned to your life. You're the only one who can look out for yourself.

Good luck and happy training!

14

Questions and Answers

Many of our television viewers write to us quite often about areas in the health-care field that are puzzling them. We feel that the answers to the questions asked might be helpful to others. Here are some of the questions most often asked.

Q. What is an **enzyme** and how important is it to digestion?

A. An enzyme is an organic substance produced in plant and animal cells which causes changes in other substances by catalytic action. To appreciate enzymes, you first have to understand that foods are chemically complex and that before your body can use them, they must be broken down into simpler forms. That's what enzymes do. Enzymes are in digestive juices, starting with saliva in the mouth. That's where carbohydrates are broken down. In the stomach, hydrochloric acid and other enzymes break down proteins, and fats are broken down with bile and still other enzymes in the small intestine. This makes enzymes very important to the digestive process.

Q. What do **assimilation** and **metabolism** mean?

A. Assimilation and metabolism are important to each other, and both are important to you. Assimilation, or absorption, is what happens after food has been digested. This digestion is usually completed in the small intestine. By that time, all foods have been broken down by enzymes into simple chemical forms, which we call nutrients. In the small intestine, those nutrients come against little fingerlike projections called villi. These contain capillaries, small blood vessels that absorb the nutrients and send them into the bloodstream. That's assimilation. The nutrients are then carried by the bloodstream to all cells

in the body. The cells use the nutrients to create energy or to build, maintain, and repair themselves. This is called metabolism.

Q. Should teenagers diet?

A. What teenagers need is not more or less food but better nutrition. With a little self-discipline and proper nutrients, teenagers can eat properly while they are growing up. If they are overweight, there is no reason why they should not be on a reducing program.

Q. Can you explain the term "friendly bacteria"?

A. Friendly bacteria are found in sour milk products such as yogurt, buttermilk, and acidophilus. These friendly bacteria balance the bad bacteria formed by waste products in the intestines. So the friendly, good bacteria help keep you clean inside.

Q. Is it advisable to drink coffee?

A. You won't gain weight on coffee, but it can interfere with the energy the body produces. Caffeine, the main ingredient in coffee, stimulates the body. That's why many people think that coffee breaks during the working day increase their energy. However, several hours after caffeine stimulates the body, the metabolism, or energy of the body, drops—sometimes to a lower level than before the coffee was drunk. So the coffee drinker drinks another cup or two, and the cycle begins again. This can be damaging to the body, especially after years of coffee drinking. The glands of the body are thrown in and out of action constantly, and the internal organs have to deal with caffeine, which is a drug. To cut down, try to drink coffee only with meals. Coffee makes digestive juices flow, and you should have solid food in the stomach for those juices to work on. The next step is to switch to decaffeinated coffee. Then cut the amount of coffee you drink. Gradually replace coffee with pro-

tein drinks—a little milk, an egg, and some protein powder will help keep your energy high throughout the day. Or if you like warm drinks, you can fix herb tea or any of the grain coffees you find in health food stores. These are foods that provide the body with nutrients it needs. Coffee has no nutrients the body needs, and it has some elements the body definitely does not need. So you don't have to quit coffee cold turkey. Just try to get into new, healthful habits.

Q. What can I do to reduce my stomach?

A. Stop putting so much garbage in it. When it comes to reducing the stomach or waistline or any other part of the body, you have to remember this physiological law: If you eat more calories or carbohydrates than your body burns for energy, the excess will be converted to fat and stored as fat.

Q. Does pulling in the stomach squash internal organs?

A. No, it may compress them a little, but it does no damage. In fact, pulling in the stomach or doing abdominal exercise is actually beneficial for internal organs.

Photo Essay

Dr. Bernie Ernst and his wife Jeanne are the co-hosts of the world-wide syndicated TV fitness show, "The Body Buddies," featuring exercise, nutrition, preventive health care, and dancercise. They may be seen on TV in virtually every city, promoting health-related products. They have been selected by several national fitness and nutritional organizations as "The Nation's Number One Fitness Couple."

About Bernie
Bernie has doctorates or advanced degrees in nutrition, Chiropractic, herbology, physiology, Natural Medicine, kinesiology, and psychology. He is a member of many health-related organizations and has won numerous awards in amateur athletics and physique contests.

About Jeanne
Jeanne was for many years the diet and weight-loss counselor at a world-famous health club and has taught exercise and dance classes. She has also won several beauty contests.

Bernie and Jeanne have co-hosted over 500 TV shows and have appeared in over 50 commercials for products in the health field.

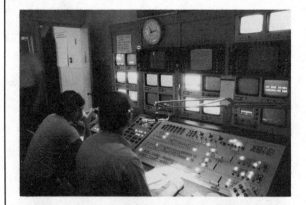

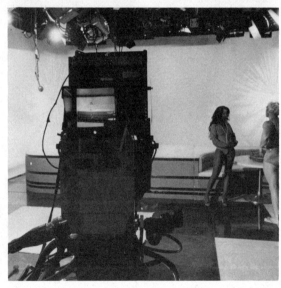

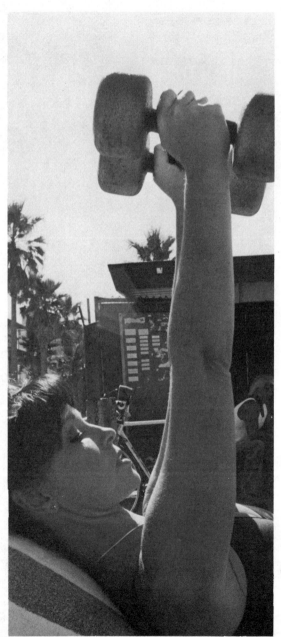

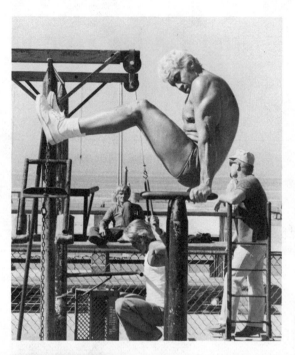

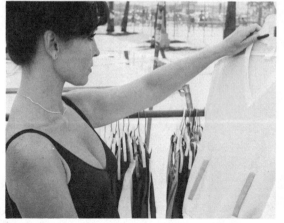

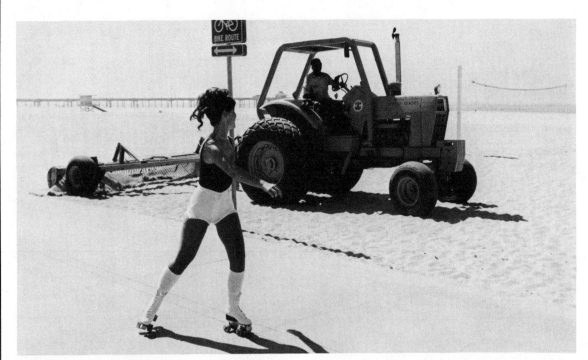

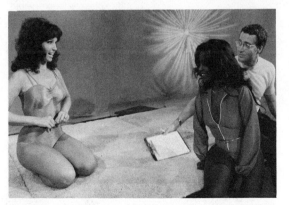

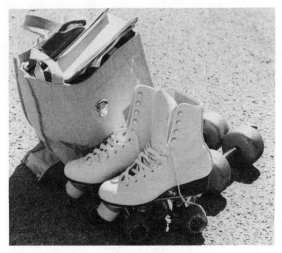

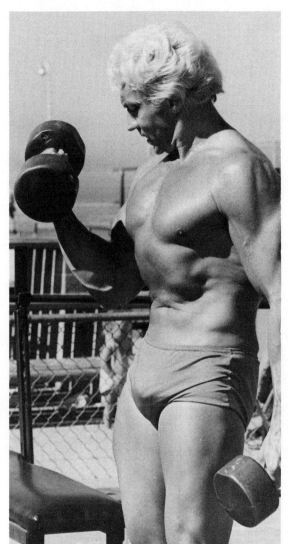

15 Photo Essay

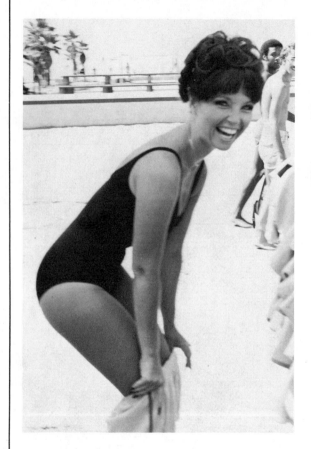

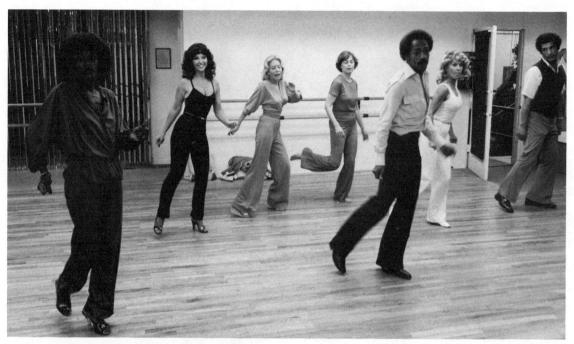

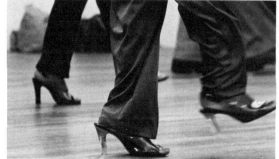

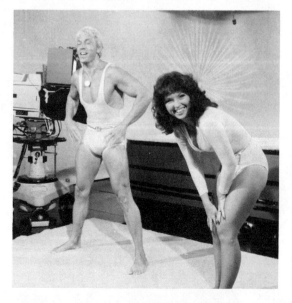

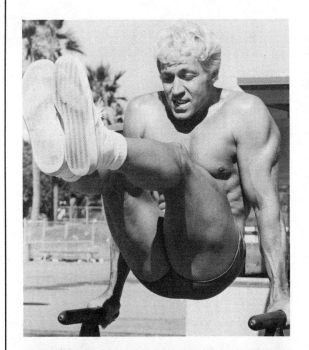

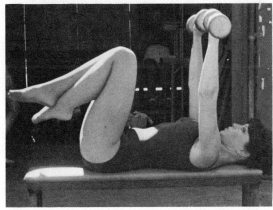

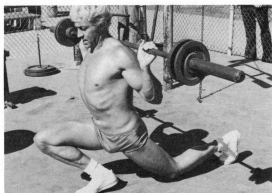

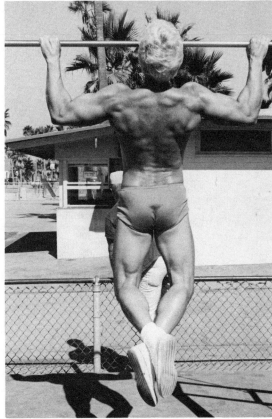

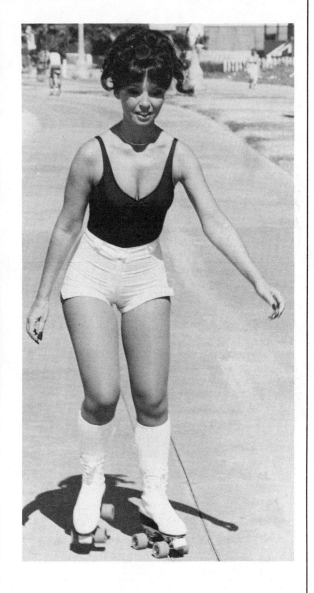